Dialogues on Human Enhancement

T0383572

We face an [illegible] gies that can be applied to our human natures with the goal of enhancing us. There are nootropic smart drugs and gene editing that influence the development of the brain. The near future promises cybernetic technologies that can be grafted onto our brains and bodies. The challenge for readers of *Dialogues on Human Enhancement* is to decide how to respond to these and other coming enhancement technologies.

As you read these dialogues you will meet passionate advocates for a variety of responses to enhancement tech, ranging from blanket rejection to ecstatic endorsement. You'll encounter Olen, for whom there is no such thing as too much enhancement. You'll meet Winston, a bioconservative who fiercely but also imaginatively opposes any human enhancement. And there is the moderate Eugenie, who strives to distinguish between enhancement technologies that should and should not be accepted. As these characters philosophically engage with each other they will benefit from the supervisory presence of Sophie, the philosopher.

Dialogues on Human Enhancement does not arrive at a single conclusion. Olen's transhumanism, Eugenie's moderation, and Winston's bioconservatism are presented as viable and necessary views as we enter a future made uncertain by human enhancement tech.

And the book also welcomes the voices of students, even – and especially – if they challenge the opinions of our age's experts. As students join the conversations in this book, they will formulate their own views about how humanity could or should be in our Age of Human Enhancement.

Nicholas Agar is Professor of Ethics at the University of Waikato in Aotearoa, New Zealand. He has written extensively on the philosophical debate about human enhancement including three books on the topic – *Liberal Eugenics* (2004), *Humanity's End* (2010), and *Truly Human Enhancement* (2013).

Philosophical Dialogues on Contemporary Problems

Philosophical Dialogues on Contemporary Problems uses a well-known form – at least as old as Socrates and his interlocutors – to deepen understanding of a range of today's widely deliberated issues. Each volume includes an open dialogue between two or more fictional characters as they discuss and debate the empirical data and philosophical ideas underlying a problem in contemporary society. Students and other readers gain valuable, multiple perspectives on the problem at hand.

Each volume includes a foreword by a well-known philosopher, topic markers in the page margins, and an annotated bibliography.

Dialogues on the Ethical Vegetarianism
Michael Huemer

Dialogues on the Ethics of Abortion
Bertha Alvarez Manninen

Dialogues on Climate Justice
Stephen M. Gardiner and Arthur R. Obst

Dialogues on Gun Control
David DeGrazia

Dialogues on Human Enhancement
Nicholas Agar

Dialogues on Free Will
Laura Ekstrom

Dialogues on Immigration and the Open Society
Chandran Kukathas

For more information about this series, please visit: www.routledge.com/Philosophical-Dialogues-on-Contemporary-Problems/book-series/PDCP

Dialogues on Human Enhancement

Nicholas Agar

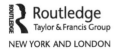 Routledge
Taylor & Francis Group

NEW YORK AND LONDON

Designed cover image: © Getty

First published 2024
by Routledge
605 Third Avenue, New York, NY 10158

and by Routledge
4 Park Square, Milton Park, Abingdon, Oxon, OX14 4RN

Routledge is an imprint of the Taylor & Francis Group, an informa business

© 2024 Nicholas Agar

ISBN: 978-1-032-34342-6 (hbk)
ISBN: 978-1-032-34225-2 (pbk)
ISBN: 978-1-003-32161-3 (ebk)

DOI: 10.4324/9781003321613

Typeset in Sabon
by KnowledgeWorks Global Ltd.

Contents

Foreword

The human enhancement project aims at making life better for us by making *us* better. Life is to be improved through the improvement of human nature. Largely inspired and fuelled by the perennial fear of ageing and death and rising frustration over the many limitations of our power and autonomy, human enhancement is meant to liberate us from the current conditions of our existence. The rapid and really quite astonishing technological advances that we have seen in the last few decades have raised hopes that it might actually be possible to escape what has long been our destiny: a life that is much shorter and often contains much more suffering than many of us would like. This is how it has always been, but now it seems that perhaps it doesn't have to stay that way. And if we *can* do something about it, why shouldn't we? Who wouldn't want a better life? Who wouldn't want to be smarter and emotionally more balanced and live a long disease-free life with their body and mind strong and undiminished by age and decay? It appears to be a no-brainer.

And yet, not everyone agrees that we should try to improve human nature, or at least not before we have thought about it more carefully. Making things better than they are is by definition good, but that doesn't tell us yet what would actually constitute an improvement. Being smarter or more intelligent than we are now certainly sounds appealing, but what exactly do we hope to gain by becoming smarter? How smart do we need to be to be able to do what we think needs doing? Will it make us happier? What does it mean to be smart anyway? Would our becoming smarter simply make it easier for us to achieve our ends, or would it also enable us to accurately identify the ends that are worth achieving? And if we are not smart enough now, how do we know that becoming smarter is indeed one of those ends?

Similar questions arise with respect to emotional enhancement and life extension. Would our lives be better if we had complete control over our emotions (and would an emotion that we can switch on and off at our will still *be* an emotion)? Or would it be best if we simply got rid of *all* emotions, on the grounds that they can only distract us from fully rational and unbiased decision-making? Or should we seek to get rid only of all "negative" or "inappropriate" emotions? But what counts as a negative or inappropriate emotion? And as for life extension, what do we need the extra time for that we would gain through the extension of our life and health span? How much longer would we want to live? Is there a cut-off point after which life would no longer be worth living, or should we aim for a potentially immortal or postmortal life?

These are just some of the questions that need to be considered before we can be certain that the kind of enhancement that we might want to pursue is actually worth having and is, as Nicholas Agar memorably called it in one of his previous books on the topic, "truly human enhancement." Things get even more complicated when we consider that, despite what Ray Kurzweil and other enhancement enthusiasts have claimed, scientific and technological progress does not seem to be governed by any reliable laws and is really quite unpredictable. Breakthroughs may happen, or they may not. They may happen now or much later or not at all. Also quite unpredictable are the consequences. We simply don't know how things will work out once human enhancement has become the order of the day and has started to change what it means to be human. Will our lives one day be "wonderful beyond imagination," as a prominent transhumanist philosopher once raved, or will we be swept out of existence by intelligent machines, which according to the same philosopher is not at all unlikely?

Nicholas Agar has been working and writing on human enhancement for more than 20 years, grappling with the many difficult and often perplexing questions it raises. And to his credit, he has never shied away from modifying his position in light of new or previously not sufficiently appreciated considerations. In his first book on the subject, *Liberal Eugenics*, published in 2004, he defended everybody's right to use enhancement technologies on themselves and their offspring in pursuit of their own personal conception of human excellence, while in his later work he has become increasingly sensitive to the dangers of all attempts to *radically* enhance humanity and suspicious of the relentlessly optimistic predictions of those who see human enhancement as a panacea for all our ills and problems.

What Agar has shown in his previous work is that it makes little sense to be for or against human enhancement. Rather, what we need to figure out is which proposed changes of our current nature are most likely to improve our lives and whether those improvements are worth the risk that we run with all changes radical enough to substantially change our lives. As Agar demonstrates in the following *Dialogues on Human Enhancement*, it is best if we do this together, by talking and listening to each other, learning what concerns others have and why they have them, and taking a variety of different viewpoints into account before we make up our minds about which concrete interventions we may want to support, and which to oppose.

Michael Hauskeller

Acknowledgements

I'm grateful to Andy Beck who invited me to write this book and shepherded it through to publication. Conversations with many friends and colleagues influenced my presentations of the book's ideas. I owe special thanks to Snita Ahir-Knight, Tracy Bowell, Bruce Curtis, Keith Dear, Rob Ferris, Stephanie Gibbons, Kiri Grant, Fabrice Jotterand, Simon Keller, Justine Kingsbury, Ed Mares, Esther Marshall, Whitney McLeod, Daniel Moseley, Michael Newall, Jonathan Pengelly, Gemma Piercy-Cameron, Arie Roskam, Ian Ravenscroft, Tayla Sanson, Vanessa Schouten, Paul Simons, Liezl Van Zyl, Mark Walker, Dan Weijers, and Furkan Yazici. I greatly benefitted from the support from and discussions of ideas with Laurianne Reinsborough, Alexei Agar, and Rafael Agar.

Introducing *Dialogues on Human Enhancement*

This is a Socratic dialogue about human enhancement. It brings the model of philosophical investigation of the ancient Greek thinker Plato to what may be the most important question about humanity's future, should we survive the climate crisis and avoid extinction by pestilential virus.

Drugs that credibly enhance some human capacities are today available in the Amazon Marketplace. These include nootropics, drugs that purport to enhance cognitive functions. Claims made on behalf of some nootropics are likely exaggerated or outright false. But there is scientific support for some of them as enhancers of human memory or powers of concentration. Recent advances in gene editing and genomics enable experimentation with DNA influencing many human traits. There are experiments in cybernetic brain implants and replacements for human body parts. I call this diverse range of interventions in human minds and bodies *enhancement technologies*.

The book presents, in the form of dialogues, a variety of views about how we should use enhancement technologies. The views advocated here range from enthusiastically embracing enhancement and all its possibilities to blanket rejection.

My inspirations for these dialogues are iconic texts for philosophers – Plato's dialogues. I have fond memories of my first exposure to philosophy through the Penguin Classics edition of Plato's *The Last Days of Socrates: Euthyphro, Apology, Crito, and*

Phaedo. Plato introduced an idea about how to conduct philosophical inquiry that came to be known as the Socratic Method – named for Socrates, the star of his dialogues. The Method is a way to seek philosophical truth by argumentative dialogue. In Plato's dialogues, characters attempt to find the truth about a variety of issues and are cajoled, coaxed, challenged, and even bullied by Socrates.

The dialogues address a variety of philosophical questions. What does it mean to enhance human cognitive and physical capacities? Should Amazon be allowed to sell drugs that may enhance human capacities in its Marketplace? Do concerns about truth in advertising require that they be described differently? What should we make of promises to use exponentially improving digital technologies to improve human capacities not just a bit, but radically? If you have consented to the application of enhancement technologies to your mind or body when does it make sense to say enough? What should we make of suggestions to rebel against our age's technological imperatives by taking our brains and bodies "off the grid"? Does the rejection of all forms of human enhancement in our technological age even make sense?

The characters in these dialogues offer a variety of answers to these and other questions about enhancement. I hope that as readers imaginatively engage with the dialogues they will venture their own answers. They should also be inspired to ask questions about human enhancement not asked in these dialogues and to consider how they might be answered.

The invitation for readers to imaginatively engage is key here. As I write in early 2023 universities are struggling to comprehend the significance of advances in generative AI, most notably from ChatGPT, the artificial intelligence chatbot developed by the American artificial intelligence research laboratory, OpenAI. ChatGPT produces work that bears many of the hallmarks of good scholarship in philosophy. Students are already submitting ChatGPT's work in their philosophy courses. There are now contributions to the academic literature written by ChatGPT.

I cannot say much in this introduction about the implications for philosophical scholarship of generative AI. I limit myself to an observation that connects the arrival of generative AI with this book's project.

   Scholars panicked by ChatGPT have tended to focus on what it cannot do. They point to the many failings of generative AI as it stands in early 2023. But these hasty responses tend to overlook the fact that generative AI is a digital technology. The former world chess champion, Garry Kasparov, has written illuminatingly about the experience of watching computers abruptly go from being mediocre players to beating the best humans.[1] It is a mistake to offer a defence of philosophy written by humans on some advantage that, though genuine in 2023, will predictably vanish with the next iterations of AI-written scholarship. The scholarship of the version of ChatGPT released in November 2022 was marred by sloppy referencing. When challenged to offer academic support for its assertions the AI hallucinated, inventing references that looked authentic but were actually to nonexistent books and articles. Generative AIs will get better at accurately citing academic literature. They are unlikely to achieve perfection, but a level of competence superior to a human scholar is surely within reach. No computer plays perfect chess. But they now play better than the best human players.

   These dialogues double down on a human advantage over machines that will be longer lasting than accurate citation of the academic literature. That is the human imagination and capacity for creativity. ChatGPT is clearly not creative. It's basically a very powerful auto-complete engine trained on 570GB of data from books, Wikipedia, and other writing from the internet.

   The thought process Friedrich Nietzsche went through to decide that "God remains dead. And we have killed him" bears little resemblance the process that ChatGPT goes through to tell you that Nietzsche "was not making a statement about the existence or non-existence of a divine being. Instead, he was making a philosophical and cultural critique of the role of religion in shaping our moral and ethical beliefs." When I ask ChatGPT to write something on the climate crisis in the style of Nietzsche it produces something that looks impressively Nietzschean to me: "For it is the Superman who shall dance upon the precipice of the abyss, resolute in his defiance against the nihilism that has engulfed the collective will of humanity." ChatGPT gives these answers because its 570GB of data contains the entirety of Nietzsche's works and many commentaries on them. It is therefore able to find much more interesting continuations than when your smartphone suggests "work" after you tap in "see you after ..."

The response of this book is to give power to the creativity that produced Nietzsche's original works. Nietzsche certainly wasn't a generative AI offering a mash-up of philosophical writing as it stood in the late nineteenth century. This book won't ask students to synthesize extracts from the vast and growing academic literature on the philosophy of human enhancement. Why attempt that when generative AI already does that so well and future generative AIs will do it even better? Instead I encourage students to think of themselves as contributing to an ongoing conversation about how technology should or shouldn't be applied to the human species. Students should imaginatively place themselves in conversation with the characters I have invented and think about what they would say. These dialogues double down on what remains humanity's superpower in this age of generative AI. Generative AIs have shown that they can convincingly fake rationality. But they cannot yet fake the human imagination. Plato's pupil Aristotle called humans the rational animal. Perhaps in this age in which rationality can so easily be simulated we need to reconceive of ourselves as the imagining animal. It's by daring acts of imagination that students will best explore the many possibilities and pitfalls of human enhancement technologies. I hope that these dialogues provoke those daring acts of imagination.

Dramatis personae for a quadrilogue on human enhancement

The four participants in these dialogues advocate a variety of views about how we should use enhancement technologies or whether we should use them at all. Olen, Eugenie, and Winston defend distinctive philosophical views about human enhancement. They should not be identified with any particular thinker. Rather their views represent broad schools of thought about how we should approach enhancement technologies.

Olen the Transhumanist: Transhumanists are the most enthusiastic supporters of human enhancement. One theme as the debate proceeds concerns *how much* enhancement humans should want. Here I understand the transhumanists as expressing a commitment not just to human enhancement, but to a great deal of it. Olen endorses *radical enhancement* – enhancement of human capacities to levels far beyond biological human norms. Transhumanists hope to see enhancement of sufficient magnitude to transform humans into different kinds of beings – posthumans. Olen finds inspiration in the rapid pace of improvement of digital technologies and aspires to apply these exponentially improving digital technologies to human nature. Olen's friends are quick to point out that some of his advocacy of enhancement is difficult to distinguish from science fiction.

Eugenie the Moderate: Olen is joined on "team enhancement" by Eugenie who supports a lesser degree of enhancement – *moderate enhancement*. Eugenie's main focus is not so much on exponentially improving digital technologies, though she certainly doesn't rule out selectively and judiciously applying them to our brains and bodies. She looks to the past, taking an idea from the Victorian polymath and cousin of Charles Darwin, Francis Galton – *eugenics*. Galton defined eugenics as the "science which deals with all influences that improve the inborn qualities of a race; also with those that develop them to the utmost advantage." In effect, Galton planned to apply to the human species the methods of selective breeding that millennia of farmers have used to improve the quality of their livestock. We can understand him as the first person to apply scientific knowledge to enhancing humanity. Galton was a brilliant mind, but his advocacy of enhancement was significantly marred by the prejudices of his age. In the popular imagination, eugenics came to be associated with other crimes of the Nazis who went farthest in the application of Galton's ideas about the scientific improvement of humanity. Eugenie learns from Galton's view but seeks to reject its most morally obnoxious implications. In her version of eugenics there will be no state-sanctioned experts who decide what kinds of lives to protect and promote and which to purge from our species. Eugenie advocates a modernization of eugenics called liberal eugenics. In this view control of humanity's future is given not to the state but to individual parents-to-be.

Winston the Bioconservative: The polar opposites of transhumanists are bioconservatives. Bioconservatives reject human enhancement. One character, Winston, defends these views. He is not a luddite, someone who seeks to reject all novel technologies. Rather Winston hopes to preserve what he views as the essence of humanity. He spends much of the discussion seeking to make apparent the many values that members of team enhancement overlook in their rush to use new scientific understanding and emerging technologies to enhance humanity.

Sophie the Philosopher: Sophie comes closest to playing the role of Socrates in these dialogues. Socrates famously joined his discussions about topics including piety, justice, and courage claiming to know nothing about the topic at hand. Sophie also disclaims knowledge about how or whether humans should enhance ourselves. She brings no view about human enhancement to the debate. Rather Sophie professes an earnest desire to learn about whether and how humans should enhance themselves. Sophie's proclaimed ignorance about the topic of the dialogue perfectly equips her to adjudicate philosophical disagreements among her friends over which is the right response to powerful enhancement technologies. She untiringly corrects her friends' many philosophical errors. But Sophie is not immune from error. Often her critiques prompt indignant responses from her friends and Sophie is forced to allow that there was more to a view than she initially dismissed.

Sophie is not a perfect fit for Socrates. In Plato's dialogues Socrates is clearly the philosophical authority – he wins all the debates in which he participates. It's fun to witness his takedowns of the good and the wise of Athens. In the *Laches* two supposed experts on courage, the distinguished generals Laches and Nicias, are exposed as intellectual fakes. They may be brave but they know much less about what it means to be courageous. Socrates' philosophical humbling of the distinguished generals is an excellent read. But the dialogue seems to leave readers with an intellectually scorched earth in which we are left with little idea about what it really means to be courageous. We finish the dialogue confident that, in spite of Socrates' entreaties to the generals to come up with new theories, he would run rings around whatever the generals come up with. In the dialogue we learn from Laches of Socrates' courage in battle. But Socrates does not draw on his brave participation in the retreat from Delium to venture his own theory about courage. We can only speculate about how Socrates the philosopher might have treated any suggestion about what it means to be courageous ventured by Socrates the brave soldier.

Sophie will challenge the philosophical views about human enhancement advanced in the dialogue, but she plays a more constructive role than Socrates does in the *Laches*. Often the other characters' views about how enhancement technologies should be applied to human nature are advanced with too much certainty. Sophie uses her superior grasp of argument to expose this philosophical overconfidence. But it's important that each of the views advanced are left standing. Readers will finish these enhancement dialogues with Olen's transhumanism, Eugenie's moderation, and Winston's bioconservatism as viable conjectures about how enhancement technologies should be applied to our brains and bodies, or whether they should be applied at all.

Put another way, the failure of these dialogues to arrive at a single winning view about enhancement is a philosophical feature not a bug. Readers should view these *Dialogues on Human Enhancement* as an essentially unfinished philosophical work. As we enter an uncertain future we will need to draw on a variety of different views about how humans could or should be. For as long as there are humans capable of applying technology to our natures we will be debating human enhancement. As we and our descendants enter the Age of Human Enhancement, we will be building on the philosophical beginnings of Olen, Eugenie, Winston, and Sophie but also adding new ideas about enhancing humans that they didn't think up.

An enhancement quadrilogue as a philosophical conversation

There are significant differences between this philosophical work on human enhancement and a conventional philosophical monograph. I have written three monographs on the human enhancement debate. There was my 2004 book *Liberal Eugenics* that defended a prerogative of prospective parents to use emerging genetic technologies to select some of the characteristics of their future children. In 2010, I published *Humanity's End* that discussed some of the philosophical excesses of those who would apply tech to our natures, radically enhancing our intellects and extending our lifespans. My human enhancement trilogy concluded with 2013's *Truly Human Enhancement* that presented a view about how much enhancement might be good for us.[2]

A philosophical monograph makes a case for a specific conclusion. It is defined by its focus and is careful to avoid extraneous material. Points are arranged to most efficiently support the intended conclusion. After a clear statement of the thesis to be defended, there's an argument that offers philosophical support for this thesis. As they make their case, good philosophers are careful to avoid extraneous or self-indulgent asides. These take up space on the page but offer no philosophical support for the view that is defended. In many philosophical monographs there is a section that responds to objections. The objections section of a monograph can cover only the merest fraction of the totality of possible responses to a thesis. But readers are meant to come out of the objections section with a sense that the author probably has a good answer to any objection they might offer. If the philosopher has done their job well, readers with dissonant views may share the sense of philosophical defeat of the distinguished generals in the *Laches*.

In my career advising students how to write essays or term papers, I have always advised that their short, say 1,500-word philosophical pieces, should adhere to the same basic structure. Good student essays need an introductory paragraph that clearly states the thesis to be defended and very concisely summarizes how the student will defend it. The argument for the thesis should be presented in the paragraphs that follow. Students should then consider and rebut objections to their view. "How many objections should I consider?" Perhaps a couple. "Can I consider only objections that are easy to rebut?" No, you should consider the objections that might be raised by an intelligent, informed opponent of your view and rebut those. A passing essay ends with a conclusion that summarizes what you accomplished in your philosophical assignment. Generative AIs are doing these traditional forms of philosophical assessment increasingly well. This should suggest the need for new forms of assessment that draw on human strengths not increasingly encroached on by machines.

In a single monograph an author is simply not permitted to change their mind. To do so is to perpetrate the greatest sin in philosophical writing, affirming a logical contradiction. Logical consistency is a requirement of the snapshot of philosophical belief presented in a monograph. If you successfully diagnose a logical contradiction in a philosophical monograph, you can cast it aside, confident that it is unworthy of your attention.

When an author has written more than one monograph on a particular topic it's possible to infer that they changed their mind on an issue of philosophical significance. Each of my three monographs on the debate about human enhancement, considered in isolation, advances a view that I maintain is logically consistent. But over twenty-five years of thinking and writing about human enhancement, I have changed my mind about some key issues. Often these changes of mind have mainly amounted to changes in emphasis.

A view which I once thought was of utmost importance, I now view as less so. I once viewed the inclusion of enhancement choices within the scope of procreative freedom as of utmost importance. That is the view presented in my 2004 book *Liberal Eugenics*. In these dialogues Eugenie advocates that view. I continue to view this as important, but less so. In consideration of the totality of implications of enhancement, I now think human enhancement can be an important expression of procreative freedom but believe that it must often be traded off against competing values.

The structure of typical philosophical conversations is quite different. While a philosophical monograph is a snapshot of the author's philosophical beliefs at a given time, a philosophical conversation occurs over time. In a monograph, the channel of information is one way. Participants in a good philosophical conversation are not only speaking, they are listening too. Good conversations are characterized by turn-taking.[3] When participants in a philosophical discussion are really listening, sometimes they change their minds. An indicator that you are actually listening is that responses to points made by your interlocutors prompt reasonable concessions from you. It's rude to just ignore the points raised by a friend and to continue with your philosophical peroration as if nothing was said. Philosophical concessions needn't be wholesale renunciations of a view. But an especially good point can necessitate significant changes in emphasis. A view formerly advanced as very important continues to be advocated but is now advanced with less confidence. This is what progress can look like over the timeframe of a philosophical conversation.

Philosophical conversations lack the strict editing of philosophical monographs. When friends get together to discuss philosophical issues they often find themselves coming back to points raised earlier. As the discussion moves on, new points are made. Sometimes it's apparent as the philosophical conversation progresses that one participant has temporarily dropped out of the discussion, only to rejoin in a way that suggests they have continued thinking about a point raised earlier and that they now feel was unfairly dismissed.

They may find that a freshly raised point has unexpected significance for an earlier issue. When they initially advanced their view they couldn't have anticipated the impact of this fresh information. They take the opportunity to double back, giving fresh expression to a point they raised earlier but now think wasn't given a fair hearing. Some of the exchanges in these dialogues get quite heated. Olen, Eugenie, Winston, and Sophie may be friends but they don't hesitate to express vigorous disagreement about how or whether at all enhancement technologies should be applied to our natures. Sometimes there is progress made on a dispute, but often the friends remain philosophically unreconciled. I think that contemporary philosophy, especially in the analytic tradition, is too characterised by argument in which on side tries their hardest to achieve the rational defeat of an adversary. We learned about the importance of that from Plato's Socrates. But an overemphasis on argument tends to occlude ways for ideas and their advocates to interact. In places in these dialogues the friends comply with the first rule of improv – "yes, and …". In an improv scene performers are encouraged to accept what has been said and build on it, rather than denying or rejecting it. In improv the first rule is intended to move a scene on in a way that encourages collaboration and creativity. Sometimes my characters comply with a philosophical first rule of improv. They don't reject an unfamiliar idea about how technologies should be applied to human nature. Rather they accept it, at least provisionally, and explore how it might be built on. At a later stage they leave themselves free to withdraw that provisional acceptance.

In philosophical conversations extraneous points are sometimes made. Discussants may briefly consider a freshly made point before collectively deciding that it is not pertinent to the issue at hand. But those passages in the record of a philosophical discussion can be valuable for readers who might have offered these points.

One of the thrills in reading Plato's dialogues as a young student is that they look like philosophical conversations. I got the impression of Plato as a young man attentively listening in on Socrates' conversations with Euthyphro, Thrasymachus, Gorgias, and the rest, frantically recording every detail of the conversations on his wax-coated wooden tablets. Of course, this is not what actually happened. The characters in Plato's dialogues are historical figures. Plato was around for some of Socrates' philosophical conversations and heard reports of many others. But being influenced by the great man didn't make Plato a mere transcriber of his insights. Plato mostly seems to treat Socrates as a vehicle for his own views.

The characters in these dialogues are my mind children. One of the great pleasures of writing these dialogues has been the opportunity to revisit my former philosophical selves and to be almost reconvinced by their reasoning. You will find evidence of my changes of mind in the views of Eugenie, Winston, and Olen. At points in my philosophical career I have supported the transhumanist thinking of Olen. I have argued for the views of the moderate Eugenie. I have advanced the criticisms of the bioconservative Winston. As I defended these views I subjected myself to the Socratic criticisms of Sophie. Viewed in the terms of my interior philosophical monologue, Sophie is the ever-present philosophical editor who hasn't hesitated to say "Nick, isn't that argument foolish!" Sophie gets to express many of the sceptical responses offered by students and colleagues over the past quarter century.

How should students read these dialogues?

If you've signed up for a philosophy course you are likely to have been driven by a sense of what matters about being human. If you find yourself wanting to respond to one of the discussants with a suggestion that they have paid insufficient attention to, then you are on the right track. The challenge for you is to give expression to this effect of enhancement that would force your chosen philosophical adversary to really pay attention. Can you invent a character, give them a brief backstory, and launch them into the debate?

As they read these dialogues students might use their characters to offer their own philosophical improvements of the conjectures and ripostes offered in the dialogues. Suppose Winston said this in response to a claim about a future enhancement tech. What should he have said? Olen gave that response. Might he have come up with something better?

Sometimes you will find points made by my characters annoying. Perhaps Olen or Winston says something that is factually erroneous or ethically outrageous. Your first instinct might be to purge that comment, to cancel it from the record of the philosophical conversation much in the way a judge in a trial will instruct a jury to ignore inadmissible evidence. Studies suggest that jurors are quite selective in their capacity to ignore evidence a judge has ruled inadmissible.[4] The best way to counter fake news in a philosophical conversation is not for discussants to do their best to collectively unhear it. This would be a near impossible feat in an emotionally heated debate about the destiny of the human species. But such claims can be countered. If Olen or Winston says something offensively wrongheaded, the best response is to invent a character who responds in ways that express your intense annoyance. Eugenie, Winston, Olen, and Sophie are friends but that won't prevent them from coming to (verbal) blows when they are advancing their different views about humanity's future. In a philosophical discussion, outrageous assertions deserve responses that are exasperated, indignant, or aggrieved. Students should empower their characters to reply to my characters' many missteps in the same fashion.

Students will notice points in the dialogues where debate seems to trail off. The philosophical debate about enhancing humans will never be over. Why not continue the dialogue? In the discussion about how to apply technology to our human natures there is always more to say. It may seem that this particular line of discussion ends with one character having the upper hand. That may be the way Sophie, Eugenie, Winston, and Olen leave it. But that's not how readers of these dialogues should. How might your character join the debate to champion the losing side?

Given that my discussants know only what I know, there are facets of the debate of which they are ignorant. There will inevitably be viewpoints about what matters, or doesn't matter, about remaining human that Sophie, Eugenie, Winston, or Olen don't consider. Perhaps readers will add their own characters to the debate. There is a limitless space of possible positions on human enhancement. The ancient Roman statesman Cicero said "There is nothing so absurd that some philosopher has not already said it." But there will be many views about the proper application of enhancement technologies to human nature unaddressed in these dialogues that are not absurd. These views may be important for our uncertain future. How would an imagined character you appoint to advance your unfairly neglected view about human enhancement engage with Sophie, Eugenie, Winston, and Olen?

I hope that the dialogue format inspires readers to take issue with points raised in the dialogues much in the way I felt motivated to respond to Socrates' too swift rebuttals of Euthyphro in that dialogue. Piety was a new concept to me but there were certainly points at which I thought Socrates was treating Euthyphro pretty poorly. The dialogue format encourages people to participate. You don't have to be an expert on an issue to offer a useful point in a discussion. Successful philosophical dialogues depend on a willingness of even the relatively uninformed to participate. Knowing less than other discussants doesn't prevent someone from usefully contributing to a philosophical conversation.

The dialogue format should encourage students to try ideas out. Students should approach the human enhancement debate with a fearless willingness to risk being wrong. If you are a young heart surgeon and want to try out your radical new idea on your next patient the consequences could be lethal. The same is not the case with novel conjectures about a future potentially made by enhancement tech. Crazy innovations can kill people in heart surgery but not in philosophy. In philosophy the worst thing that can happen to you is suffering the opprobrium of your colleagues in a department seminar.

As we will see, even the experts are often wrong about the future. A mistaken student idea about future enhancement tech is likely to do less harm than an institutionally empowered expert's mistakes about the future.

My characters make some claims with conviction. But in other cases they are less committed to the views they advance. They seem to be advancing conjectures and are happy to retract and try something new when their friends put up too much philosophical resistance. This is a feature of good philosophical conversations that sadly does not carry over to philosophers' polished published thoughts. I invite students to be guided by this ethos when they add their voices to the dialogues. Perhaps there is a perspective on the enhancement debate that they want to air, but do not want to advocate as their own view. Why not invent a character and have them try the view out on your behalf?

The dialogue format suggests new ways to assess philosophy students. Rather than assigning a term paper, students might be challenged to contribute novel points to a dialogue. The debate between Eugenie and Winston on eugenics concludes this way. How should it have continued? Here's a section from the discussion on performance-enhancing drugs in athletics and chess. Which new characters and viewpoints will the student add to that section to philosophically improve it? Could you add 1,000 words of dialogue, either using my existing characters or with new characters that would do justice to a philosophical issue that my characters neglect?

Philosophical conversations are naturally interdisciplinary

This is a philosophical work but the fact that it is a conversation lends itself to interdisciplinary contributions. My characters come from different disciplines. Sophie anticipates a future in academic philosophy. The real-world counterparts of Olen the tech entrepreneur, Eugenie the public servant, and Winston the historian would never write for a philosophy journal. But when they make points in a philosophical conversation their suggestions and objections do not come with an asterisk signalling that they are philosophical outsiders and their points can be safely ignored. It would be simple rudeness to neither hear a criticism nor be curious about what is behind it.

We've heard that a fast-changing world demands different kinds of courses and research from universities. The traditional academy's specializations were a great fit for the predictable needs of the economies that emerged from the Second Industrial Revolution.[5] But they've been seriously wrong-footed by the digital revolution, climate change, and the pandemic.

These issues are addressed by the traditional academy. You can take philosophy courses on the ethics of climate change. A challenge for these courses is the mismatch between what their titles promise – a broad focus on the climate crisis that gives equal hearing to what climate scientists, economists, sociologists, philosophers, and so on, say – and what they provide which is a philosopher's take on what specialists from other disciplines say in which there is typically no right of reply. In a philosophy course you might expect a few students who have done some economics, but you are unlikely to find an economics professor in your audience.

If we were reinventing universities from scratch now, what we call interdisciplinary courses would surely exist in their own right. There would be disciplines that pull together all the different kinds of knowledge that bear on humanity's response to climate change or the issue of what kinds of societies could emerge from the pandemic. But we are stuck with the research and teaching priorities of the traditional university. Emerging issues such as the future of work in the digital economy find themselves awkwardly shoehorned into philosophy, sociology, or economics courses.

Must conversations that welcome the contributions of outsiders be academically shallow? The ideal academic work on the future of work in the digital economy will number well in excess of 100,000 pages permitting it to give exemplary coverage of the contributions of all the many disciplines – economics, labour studies, anthropology, sociology, psychology, cognitive science, computer science, political science, philosophy, and so on. Interdisciplinary teams could write such a work, but even they face the obstacle of disciplinary scholars brought together for workshop who can't really give proper weight in the contributions of scholars from other disciplines. I propose that effective interdisciplinary discussions compensate for a lack of disciplinary depth with an increase in breadth. When an interdisciplinary scholar makes a point about the ethical consequences of automation, they must demonstrate awareness of the diversity of views across the academy. It can be tempting for a philosopher to simplify the views of economists – "Economists all follow John Maynard Keynes in viewing technological unemployment as painful but temporary." I might get away with that in a paper presented to an audience of philosophers or submitted to an academic philosophy journal. But I doubt that an audience that included people who have taken courses in economics would let me get away with it.

Penalties for interdisciplinary teaching are reinforced by penalties for interdisciplinary research. There is a regrettable citation penalty for papers that draw on research from distant fields.[6] This means that there is little incentive for economists to care much about what philosophers say about the future of work – or vice versa. If we publish in our own discipline's journals, we are unlikely to be pulled up for errors about disciplinarily distant scholarship.

This is a philosophical debate so its experts reside in philosophy departments and their points are mainly made in philosophy texts. It goes without saying that philosophers are the experts on the philosophy of human enhancement. Someone entirely untrained in philosophy could probably not write a passing term paper on the ethics of enhancement, still less have an article accepted for publication in a philosophy journal. But the dialogue format welcomes suggestions from elsewhere. You may not be able to write a passing philosophy term paper but you surely can make a valuable contribution to a philosophical conversation about applying enhancement technologies to humans.

A quadrilogue at the outset of the Age of Human Enhancement

These *Dialogues on Human Enhancement* are timely. We are entering what I will call the Age of Human Enhancement. This Age of Human Enhancement isn't limited to a future when enhanced beings walk among the unenhanced human leftovers. The Age doesn't begin with the arrival of the superheroes and supervillains of Marvel and Amazon's series *The Boys*. It commences when we have enhancement technologies that credibly enhance some human capacities. If you visit the Amazon Marketplace you will find compounds sold as enhancers of human powers of memory or concentration. Today's enhancement technologies certainly don't grant unpowered flight or eyes that sprout laser beams. But they could constitute the first steps toward a future in which humans do have those powers.

Discussions of human enhancement technologies address an essentially uncertain future. The participants present conjectures about the development of future technologies that may not come to pass. Suppose the friends were to reconvene in 2043 to discuss the philosophy of human enhancement. The dialogue should be very different indeed. Olen especially draws on forecasts about how digital technologies will advance and how they may be applied to our natures. Perhaps when the friends meet in 2043 they will find that Olen's forecasts have been confirmed. If so, Olen may feel vindicated. But he should still listen to Winston's view that this embrace of enhancement was mistaken. Perhaps in 2043 they will find that few of Olen's forecasts have come to pass. This will not falsify Olen's transhumanism. But, at a minimum, it will call for his claims to be significantly revised.

One of the themes of these dialogues is the way the Age of Human Enhancement requires a change in focus by philosophers. Some of the disagreements between Eugenie, Winston, Sophie, and Olen concern how the arrival of technologies that plausibly enhance human traits, with the promise of more powerful enhancement technologies over the coming years, should change the way we talk about human enhancement.

Prior to the Age of Human Enhancement, philosophers presented thought experiments that addressed the very idea of using technology to enhance humans. These thought experiments were informative about the overall moral acceptability of using technology to enhance human traits. But the focus of philosophers on idealized enhancement technologies can obscure the detail of the techs that we are beginning to apply to our natures. A philosopher may advance a persuasive thought experiment about an enhancement pill that, once swallowed, grants a millennial lifespan. This may show that the very idea of extending human lifespans is not morally mistaken. A problem with the fantastical enhancers of philosophers' thought experiments, as we enter the Age of Human Enhancement, is that they can distract attention from the details of the actual inventions coming to the Amazon Marketplace. Too many technologically idealized stories make it difficult to appropriately balance the potential benefits brought by enhancement technologies against their moral and prudential costs. Advice informed by the scientific detail of enhancement technologies should guide the tradeoffs demanded by the Age of Human Enhancement. Put another way, if the debate about human enhancement was once purely philosophical, in the Age of Human Enhancement it must be interdisciplinary. Philosophers have essential roles in these interdisciplinary conversations. Our command of reason means that we are ideally qualified to adjudicate the debates between technologists, historians, and economists about how our species should enter the Age of Human Enhancement.

Among the more scandalous philosophical conjectures of the bioconservative Winston is the suggestion that the philosophers who use fantastical thought experiments to advocate enhancement have, knowingly or not, been co-opted by commercial interests that expect to be selling us increasingly powerful enhancement technologies in the years to come. The profits from the first safe enhancement technologies proven to significantly boost human cognitive powers could be enormous. This means that what looks like philosophy is actually marketing copy. I would be curious to see how students choose to engage with or continue the sections of the dialogues in which Winston advances this view.

Our time of overconfident experts

Philosophers need advice from other experts as we enter the Age of Human Enhancement. But we must be careful about how we listen to that advice.

The aspect of Plato's Socrates that these dialogues most celebrate is not the Socrates who wins every argument, but the Socrates of the *Apology* who says "I neither know nor think I know" (in Plato, *Apology* 21d). This is the Socratic Paradox, often expressed as "I know that I know nothing." In spite of this proclaimed ignorance Socrates readily defeats philosophical adversaries who claim to know a great deal. Philosophers tend to focus on the contradictory nature of the Paradox – how can you know that you know nothing if you really know nothing? But in our time of experts we most need philosophers empowered to challenge the assertions of experts, even if they accept that they know less.

We have needed experts to help us navigate the pandemic. They informed us about the value of vaccines and how best to take them. Over the next years we will need to listen more attentively to the advice of climate experts on how best to slow the changes to our planet initiated by the Industrial Revolution.

There are many experts rushing to offer advice about the proper use of enhancement technologies. We need this advice too. But we must be wary of expert advice about humanity's future offered with too much confidence. A Socratic questioner must question all overconfident forecasts about an essentially uncertain future.

When we look back at a decade of unpleasant surprises there has all too often been an overconfident expert encouraging us to proceed into an essentially uncertain future with scant regard for what could happen if things don't go exactly according to plan. It can be dangerous to enter the future with an overconfident sense of what it will bring. As I write these words the world is – fingers crossed – emerging from the COVID-19 pandemic. But we have seen too many overconfident forecasts of an imminent end to the pandemic.

Since the debate about human enhancement is about the future we should learn from the political scientist Philip Tetlock what constitutes good forecasting.[7] Tetlock highlights the incentives for overconfident simplifications of what we can say about future events. Tetlock's term is "dress to impress forecasting." He points to the increasing risk of this error about the future when an expert finds themselves marketing a book on TV. TV watchers and book buyers are part of the problem. As we enter a frightening future, we like experts who confidently tell us how it's going to be. We buy their books and crave their soundbites. Sophie will take a Socratic approach when she challenges the overconfident statements of the members of team enhancement about the future that enhancement technologies could make.

You might ask what's wrong with a bit of overconfident optimism as we hopefully emerge from the pandemic. Isn't it good to enthuse about a future in which enhancement technologies delete the human frailties that allowed the millions of deaths of the pandemic? Perhaps. But we mustn't forget that it was unchecked optimism, specifically about our technologies, that set us up for this. The Harvard scientist Steven Pinker's book *Enlightenment Now* decried the pessimism about progress that seemed to have taken root in many circles, especially in the academy. Pinker sought to dispel this negativity – "here is a shocker: The world has made spectacular progress in every single measure of human well-being. Here is a second shocker: Almost no one knows about it." According to Pinker there's much better to come. In his celebration of progress Pinker offers an aside about disease outbreaks – "advances have made humanity more resilient to natural and human-made threats: disease outbreaks don't become pandemics."[8] Pinker's book was published in 2018. Pinker wasn't claiming to be an expert on pathogens or epidemiology. But we can ask to what extent his confidence about the power of progress set some of the most technologically advanced nations up for their high death tolls from COVID-19.

The spirt of Socrates in this debate about human enhancement and its future is best represented by Sophie's willingness to challenge the overconfident claims of her friends. Perhaps Olen will turn out to be right about the power of exponentially improving digital technologies to reshape human nature for the better. But at this early stage in the Age of Human Enhancement we need Sophie to correct his overconfidence.

I hope students are inspired by this. If the enhancement debate is really a debate about humanity's future and even the experts can get the future wrong then perhaps your speculations are no less worthy of consideration than theirs.

Notes

1 Kasparov, Garry, *Deep Thinking: Where Machine Intelligence Ends and Human Creativity Begins* (PublicAffairs, 2017).
2 Agar, Nicholas, *Liberal Eugenics: In Defence of Human Enhancement* (John Wiley & Sons, 2004), Agar, Nicholas, *Humanity's End: Why we should Reject Radical Enhancement* (MIT Press, 2010), Agar, Nicholas, *Truly Human Enhancement: A Philosophical Defense of Limits* (MIT Press, 2013).
3 Stivers, Tanya, N. J. Enfield, Penelope Brown, Christina Englert, Makoto Hayashi, Trine Heinemann, Gertie Hoymann, et al., "Universals and cultural variation in turn-taking in conversation", *Proceedings of the National Association of Sciences*, 106(26), 2009.
4 Kassin, S. M. and S. R. Sommers, "Inadmissible testimony, instructions to disregard, and the jury: Substantive versus procedural considerations", *Personality and Social Psychology Bulletin*, 23(10), 1997.
5 Davidson, Cathy, *The New Education: How to Revolutionize the University to Prepare Students for a World in Flux* (Basic Books, 2017).
6 Yegros-Yegros, Alfredo, Ismael Rafols, and Pablo D'Este, "Does Interdisciplinary Research Lead to Higher Citation Impact? The Different Effect of Proximal and Distal Interdisciplinarity", *PLoS ONE*, 10(8), 2015.
7 Tetlock, Philip and Dan Gardner, *Superforecasting: The Art and Science of Prediction* (Crown Publishers, 2015).
8 Pinker, Steven, *Enlightenment Now: The Case for Reason, Science, Humanism, and Progress* (Viking, 2018).

Night 1   What should we say about gene-edited twins who may have been enhanced?

Meeting at the Filthy Spoon Café

Winston is sitting at a table drinking coffee. Eugenie arrives, seating herself across from him.

Eugenie: Winston! So good to see you after all these years. It seems like you got that anonymous email invitation too.

Winston: Yes. It's good to see you too. But ... I'm sorry to report that the coffee here hasn't gotten any better.

Eugenie: (*takes a sip of her newly purchased coffee*) Actually, I quite like this. The smelly socks aspect brings back memories of all those times we got together and engaged in intense debate about the issues of the day. Remember our resolution some twenty years ago to take immediate action on climate change. That was binding on us, but sadly not on any politicians. Wasted words those might have been, but the pleasure of debating them somehow excused any amount of bad coffee and poorly mixed cocktails.

Winston: I was surprised get the invitation too. I'm guessing you remember Olen and Sophie – they seem to have been invited too.

Olen and Sophie arrive and seat themselves at the table.

Sophie: Welcome back to the Filthy Spoon! I should own up to the fact that I'm the one who invited you. I'm glad the

DOI: 10.4324/9781003321613-1

anonymous invitation intrigued you all enough to turn up. People are so busy these days and I was worried that if I didn't make it seem mysterious you wouldn't turn up. I'm confident that the mix of minds we have around this table brings sufficient diversity to make progress on what I think is the most pressing problem of our age.

Olen: (*groans*) I hope that this isn't going to be yet another lecture on climate change and how we really must be doing so much more about it.

Sophie: Climate change clearly belongs at the top of our collective agenda. But if anything, this is more important. I'm interested in category of technologies that we are beginning to apply to our natures to enhance our abilities. These enhancement technologies used to be the stuff of science fiction. But now they are happening.

Winston: That does sound important, though I do question your suggestion that it is a more important issue that human-caused climate change that is already bringing misery to millions and is likely to get worse.

Sophie: That's a good point Winston. In the wide-ranging discussion that we will have there will be plenty of opportunity to ask questions about the relative philosophical importance of the debates about climate and human enhancement. I know this many seem like we are about to start a student tutorial, but can each of us introduce ourselves and catch up on what we've been doing since we were last here all those years ago? Winston, can you go first?

Winston: I've just gotten a tenure-track job in the History Programme at our alma mater. I'm preparing classes and finishing a book for Routledge on etiquette and manners in the ancient Rome of the late Republic. This debate about human enhancement is new to me. Sci-fi really isn't my thing! You'll remember that I used to sit out your *Star Trek* viewing marathons. I'm looking forward to our discussion and I feel a sense of fascination about what you'll all say. I'm open to changing my mind as our discussion progresses. But here's my historian's take on the human enhancement debate. We shouldn't overlook the line of the American philosopher George Santayana that "Those who do not learn history are doomed to repeat it." I think a related issue arises in respect of the things we care about. Those who don't adequately reflect on the values gifted to us by our histories risk harming them from applying shiny new technologies willy-nilly to our natures.

Olen: Good luck with the staid miseries of academia, Winston. I can't say that I envy you. But I'm sure you've all been following my progress. That social media idea that I used to nag you all about at this very table has become a unicorn, which, for the uninitiated, is a company with a valuation of one billion dollars without being listed on the stock market. At least, it's not listed yet. We launch publicly next week. I'll be taking the opportunity to show off some of the company's thrilling tech to you guys. You won't be surprised to hear that I'm much more enthusiastic about improving our natures by applying powerful technologies to them. Like Winston I'm open to changing my mind as the discussion progresses. I may be a tech dude rather than a philosopher, so I know nothing about philosophical debates about human enhancement, but I do know quite a lot about progress in digital technologies. I predict amazing things as we increasingly apply exponentially improving digital technologies to our natures. We need to give more power to individuals working hardest to develop these technologies. I'm confident that an unhindered free market in enhancement technologies will turn out for the best. If we want to achieve the best outcomes for humanity we do best to follow the money.

Sophie: Still the same old Olen I see, but perhaps a bit richer.

Olen: Winston, I'm not sure how you're surviving on that meagre academic salary of yours. But if you can scrape together some cash to invest, you could more than make up for some mistaken career choices. (*Winks at Winston.*) That offer applies to you too, Eugenie and Sophie. What have you been doing with yourselves since our last Filthy Spoon debate? If I remember accurately it was more of philosophical brawl about the morality of travelling to Nicaragua to support the Contras than a polite debate.

Eugenie: I ended up working for government. One of the benefits of spurning the academic path is that I have more money to invest than Winston. I'm interested to hear more about your tech start-up, Olen. I'm also interested in hearing more about these enhancement technologies. There's an essential role for government here. I don't think we should be looking to individuals to solve the problem of climate change. Companies see profit in products marketed as good for the environment, but my view is that free market solutions to climate change will always fall short. I think the solution must come from democratically elected governments. I'm new to this debate about human enhancement but my starting view is that if we are all to benefit from enhancement technologies, government will need to take charge. Let's ensure that we make these powerful technologies available as broadly as possible.

Olen: Eugenie, it sounds like you and I are going to be allies in the philosophical debate about human enhancement. Our disagreements will be about the role of government. From my tech perspective, government stifles innovation. It may be the case that the rich get powerful enhancement techs first. But there's a pattern, especially apparent in digital technologies. These techs quickly get cheaper.

Eugenie: This sounds a bit too much like trickle-down economics to me. Olen, are you oblivious to the challenge of wealth inequality that free markets aggravate?

Sophie: This does sound like an issue we will need to address. But first I should bring you up to speed on my progress.

It took a while for me to find myself vocationally. After a few false starts, I came back to university and enrolled in a PhD programme in philosophy.

Olen: Ahh ... someone else who wants to be poor for the rest of her life. Perhaps I could make an investment in my company on your behalf.

Sophie: Thanks, but no thanks. I should reveal an ulterior motive in inviting you here. I've decided to write my PhD thesis on this topic. I thought back over our conversations and decided that another discussion with you all would be a great way for me to get started. Olen, I've learned about the importance of impartiality as a philosopher. I strongly suspect that, with your tech interests, you will be advocating a view about humanity's future that I should disagree with.

Eugenie: This sounds like fun. (*Olen and Winston nod enthusiastically.*)

The He Jiankui affair

Sophie: Perhaps I can get the ball rolling by discussing a particular case that I came across in the media. I wonder if it caught your attention. (*Sophie brings out her tablet and clicks on a link. There is a news item about the Chinese scientist He Jiankui.*)

He Jiankui was imprisoned in China for using gene editing technology to edit the genomes of twin girls, given the pseudonyms Lulu and Nana. The stated goal of He Jiankui's experiment was to cause a mutation in a gene that makes a protein HIV uses to get into human cells. Lulu and Nana's father was HIV-positive and the plan was to protect the girls from infection by deactivating the gene. He Jiankui deliberately avoided the oversight that would have been offered by ethics committees on experiments in human reproductive technology.

Sophie: I think you'll all remember the stories about this case.

Eugenie: I do remember the story. I have to say that I'm on He Jiankui's side in this. Yes, he did break some rules. But if we can use the technological breakthrough of gene editing to protect future generations from HIV then I'm all in favour. Perhaps he goes to jail now. But if all goes well then perhaps in a couple of decades' time he will be getting his Nobel prize for contributions toward a disease-free future for humanity. Sometimes silly rules have to be broken for the betterment of humanity.

Olen: Hurray for that! I bring good news from the world of digital technology. Fast-developing digital techs promise disease therapies that will soon make He Jiankui's approach look pretty primitive. I'm betting on a future with digital technologies that treat and prevent HIV much better than anything He Jiankui did for Lulu and Nana.

Winston: Sorry to press the pause button on your tech hype, Olen, but can we at least reflect on what it will be like to be them? They are going to have to grow up as experimental beings. I can only imagine the internet sleuths of twenty-years' time who've decided to find them and reveal their identities to the world just to satisfy our curiosity about whether their edited genome might have turned them blue. From what I'm reading here, He Jiankui didn't really think much about them. He just wanted the accolades of being the first scientist to create gene-edited human beings. But I'm wondering what this has to do with your thesis topic, Sophie. Were Lulu and Nana enhanced? It looks to me like the scientist just wanted to ensure that they had a start to their lives free of HIV. He Jiankui was reckless, but his goal, though not his means, seems morally acceptable to me. I'm wondering what this has to do with the debate about human enhancement. You don't have to be enhanced to live without HIV.

Sophie: Thanks Winston. One of our first orders of business must be to define human enhancement. But I've only told half the story about He Jiankui and Lulu and Nana. The gene that he deleted was CCR5. This deletion may have had another, somewhat unexpected, effect. And no, I doubt that it turned their skin blue.

Olen: Go on! The suspense is killing me.

Sophie: There's a phenomenon known as pleiotropy in which a single gene affects two or more seemingly unrelated traits. Scientists have discovered that a surprising number of human genes affect the development of the brain. A gene-editing experiment on mice suggests that the deletion of CCR5 may improve the ability to form new memories and learn. Now, I understand that there are differences between humans and mice, but both species are mammals so we should be open to the possibility that an effect on the mouse brain might carry over to deletion of the gene in humans.

Olen: I'm clearly going to be the science guy in this discussion. I certainly look forward to telling you all about some of the possibilities that may come from applying new technologies to our human natures. But I should caution you that the research you are referring to is highly speculative. Further research on CCR5 may disconfirm the connection between the edit and cognitive enhancement.

Sophie: There will be debate about the facts of this case. Perhaps we can consider it as a philosophical thought experiment. Let's seriously consider the possibility that an edit that may offer some protection against HIV also improves memory and learning. That way we will be prepared for a future in which it does.

Eugenie: Did He Jiankui say anything about this possible effect on Lulu and Nana?

Sophie: He did. He said "I saw that paper, it needs more independent verification. I am against using genome editing for enhancement."

Winston: That sounds very suspicious to me. It seems to make it far too easy for a reckless scientist to tamper with the human genome and to disavow any awareness of ill effects. How can that philosophically cagey statement possibly justify applying tech in need of "more independent verification" to human beings?

Sophie: Well, he did have the stated goal of protecting the twins from HIV. That seems like a morally worthy therapeutic aim. I'm thinking that we will need to revisit the relationship between therapeutic use of techs like gene editing and using them to enhance. But for the time being let's put that issue to one side. There's a philosophical principle that seems to be behind He Jiankui's apparent lack of concern that his intervention might have enhanced the twins. It's the Doctrine of Double Effect. According to one version of the Doctrine it is sometimes permissible to cause a harm as a double effect – or side effect – of doing something good. This is so even though it would not be permissible to cause such a harm as a means to bringing about the same good end.

Eugenie: This seems to justify He Jiankui's disregard for effects on the twins beyond possible protection against HIV. Possible effects on intelligence are just a side effect of achieving the good end of protecting against HIV. Effects on intelligence weren't means to keeping the virus out of their cells.

Winston: That's such a scam! The Doctrine makes it too easy for scientists to experiment on enhancing human cognitive abilities in a way that dodges ethical evaluation. If so, many genes that affect the brain's development are pleiotropic – they can always say that they were really trying to do something else and only incidentally enhancing.

Olen: I can't believe that I'm saying this. But I strongly agree with Winston. The Doctrine of Double Effect is pretty foolish. If I drop a bomb on your house am I excused from worrying about the double effect of killing its occupants just because my stated intention was a cool fireworks display. Of course, I strongly disagree with Winston about the goal of human enhancement. But I strongly assert that scientists should be open about what we are trying to do. We should be celebrating Lulu and Nana's possible cognitive enhancement rather than pretending it was an accident.

Sophie: There's more to the Doctrine of Double Effect, Olen. But getting into that might distract us from our proper focus. The fact that you and Winston agree about the Doctrine and disagree about human enhancement suggests that it's not really what matters philosophically here.

The importance of being reasonable about an essentially uncertain future

Winston: I see the benefits of your philosophical training already, Sophie, quick-marching us back on track to the debate about human enhancement. So, as the philosopher, can you offer some guidance about how we are supposed to conduct our discussion?

Sophie: I have fond memories of the intense debates we used to have. We've all grown up a bit since then and we've significantly cut back on our drinking. One of the things that I remember about the effects of alcohol on our debates is that the longer the discussion went, the more we would drink, and the louder our voices became. By the end of our evenings we were basically shouting at each other. I remember that there was a tendency for those who shouted the loudest to believe that they were winning the debate. I'm not looking at anyone in particular ... Olen. Can we agree to a no shouting rule?

Olen: Thanks Sophie ... a not especially subtle reference to my youthful argumentative enthusiasm. But I think I have a fix for your no alcohol suggestion that should make everyone happy.

Sophie: I can't wait to hear it. But I have another suggestion about how we should conduct our discussion. I love philosophy. But I do find that philosophers sometimes have a problem with being overconfident in their assertions. They love debating, perhaps too much. When they get into these debates the testosterone starts flowing and they want desperately to be the winner of the debate.

Olen: Killjoy ...

Sophie: Philosophical overconfidence is a big problem when we are talking about enhancement. We are talking about an uncertain future. The gene-editing technologies that we've just been discussing are recent inventions. We can make educated guesses about future technologies that we may apply to our natures but it would be foolish to say that we can predict the future for sure. There's so much we have yet to learn. Let's not be too overconfident in our claims about the technologies we may someday apply to our natures.

Olen: So I'm not allowed to be very enthusiastic about the wonderful future that can come from applying fast-advancing technologies to our quite backwards human nature? I hope you all appreciate that the last big hardware upgrade on us came in the Pleistocene, a geological epoch that that started about 2.5 million years ago and ended about 12,000 years ago. Biologically speaking, humans have been essentially unchanged since then. We've been doing our best with brains and bodies that worked well when we were hunting and foraging but can't be expected to sustain us into an increasingly technological future. Humanity so badly needs a hardware upgrade. We're pushing this Pleistocene biological tech beyond its limits.

Winston: Sophie, can you remind Olen that this is a philosophical discussion. We've heard about his social media unicorn. But does his introduction of this tech-speak really help here?

Olen: Thanks Winston. I can tell that you and I are going to be adversaries for much of this discussion. All I ask is that you open your mind to some of the possibilities opened up by new technologies, especially digital ones. Perhaps a hardware upgrade would address the problem of too many people who can't see that vaccines can offer protection against a killer virus, or that there is a connection between our carbon emissions and climate change. I remember that the ancient Greek philosopher defined humans as the rational animals. But these glitches in our rationality strongly suggest that we could be improved. Look to digital technologies for those improvements!

Sophie: You've made your view apparent, Olen. I think it's important that you argue for it enthusiastically. But I want you to listen to the views of Winston and Eugenie, even if you disagree with them. That's part of what it means to be reasonable. We have a historian here. I think he might offer some philosophical context for confident claims that technology will fix our biggest problems.

Winston: We can be a bit gullible when smart people offer exciting forecasts about an essentially uncertain future. I think there are patterns more apparent to people who study history than to those overly focused on shiny tech. I read Siddhartha Mukherjee's 2010 book about the war on cancer – *The Emperor of All Maladies*. It documents a history of confident forecasts of imminent cures for cancer. Many of them delivered better cancer therapies but the forecast cure for cancer didn't arrive. I think we should keep these disappointments in mind as we hear about your exciting enhancement techs. It's easy to make exciting promises, but harder to deliver on them. That's an important lesson from history.

Sophie: These are good points. I think I can see how to introduce rational doubts about the future of enhancement tech into our conversations.

Olen: OK ... I guess.

Sophie: Olen, this really isn't boring pedantry. Think of it as an appropriate epistemic modesty. One of my philosophical heroes, Socrates, has a paradox named for him – the Socratic Paradox. Rendered approximately, he said, that the only thing he knew was that he knew nothing.

Olen: Ha! How can he know that, then?

Sophie: You've caught on to the Paradox! But I prefer to view it as a farsighted expression of epistemic modesty. Ancient Athens was full of people claiming to know things that they actually didn't. Socrates didn't need to pretend that he knew anything to prove that they didn't know what they claimed to know.

Olen: Philosophers eh ...

Sophie: Socrates' warning is especially important to bear in mind as we approach an uncertain future.

Winston: Yes Sophie. That's a very important point to raise. I can I add a point that wouldn't have been apparent to Socrates. That is the role of money in forecasts offered by people in tech. Yes ... I'm looking at you, Olen. Mark Zuckerberg got rich offering us a future in which Facebook would bring everyone in the world closer together. What happens we collectively offer the same trust to those who offer to sell us technologies that will remake our human natures?

Sophie: I think we are off to an excellent start with our philosophical investigation of human enhancement. We have a good many questions and speculations – a great way to start a discussion about an uncertain future.

I propose that we meet again over several evenings to really get to the bottom of this enhancement thing, philosophically speaking. I hope you've understood the ground rules for our discussion. I think we should meet again at the Filthy Spoon tomorrow evening to continue our philosophical investigation. I think tomorrow we should attend to the first philosophical order of business which will be to work out what we really mean by human enhancement. The term "enhancement technologies" has been bandied about a bit. What does it include?

Winston: Apparently, it may include gene-editing technologies.

Sophie: Yes, but I want to do better than just giving an example.

Eugenie: Excellent, let's meet again at the Filthy Spoon for some terrible coffee and philosophical enlightenment.

Doing philosophy in the Metaverse!

Olen: I think we can do better than that.

Winston: Go on.

Olen: Let's meet geographically in the Filthy Spoon … but really in the virtual reality of the Metaverse.

Eugenie: Olen, I'm not sitting here with a virtual reality headset on just to avoid seeing the Filthy Spoon's tasteless decor. Also, I don't see how it would make the coffee taste any better.

Olen: I have a fix for that. Winston, I'm surprised that in your conspiracy theorizing about the future of human enhancement you didn't mention Elon Musk. He's my hero and definitely the man with the clearest vision about how tech can make a better world. He's going to use tech to fix climate change, and failing that he will relocate us to Mars. The good news is that Musk is now applying his genius to our human natures.

Eugenie: How is this going to help us to better understand the philosophy of human enhancement?

Olen: What if I could set you up with some very impressive digital enhancement technology designed by Musk's company Neuralink. Neuralink produces implantable brain-machine interfaces that can enhance the reach of our minds. Would that convince you of the power of digital enhancement tech?

Sophie: We're listening …

Olen: I've brought along some of the tech that Musk's com-
               pany has produced. Here are some prototype neural
               laces. They can take information from the world and
               present it directly to our brains. We could set them up
               to relay information about the Filthy Spoon which is
               where we will physically be. But we could set it up to
               convey the sights and sounds of pretty much anywhere.
               Sophie, I think you said you wanted to discuss defini-
               tions of enhancement at our next meeting. I've thought
               of the perfect virtual locale. If each of us has a neural
               lace we can all meet there and continue our discussion.

Winston: This does sound absurd. Surely there's a catch.

Olen: Hmm, yes. There will be a teensy neurosurgical
               procedure.

Eugenie: (*shouts*) WHAT!?

Olen: Don't worry, Eugenie. It's entirely reversible and certi-
               fied safe by Musk and his elite tech people. Why don't I
               make it worth your while by clarifying that this consti-
               tutes a test of a very interesting prototype variant of the
               neural lace. You will all be appropriately remunerated
               with stock in Tesla, Inc.

Winston: There's no way I'm going to let you slice into my brain
               just so you can make your bad argument for enhance-
               ment seem hyperreal.

Olen: You can view it as an enhancement version of try-before-
               you-buy. Sophie, unless we get to see what digital tech
               can do the discussion will be hamstrung by Winston's
               prejudices.

Sophie: In the interests of philosophical truth, I'm prepared
               to try it. I think that you all know that I am diabetic
               and I use some digital technology – an insulin pump –
               to regulate my blood sugar. Perhaps there's no big
               difference between my prosthetic pancreas and this
               neuroprosthesis.

Eugenie: Let's give it a go then.

Winston: This is all a bit reminiscent of *The Matrix*. Olen, are you pretending to be Morpheus and offering us the choice between the Blue and Red pills? It looks like we are choosing the Red pill and going into philosophical wonderland to see how deep the human enhancement rabbit hole goes. I'm pretty confident that this will be a big mistake, but OK.

Night 2 Enhancement technologies, doping athletes, and the meaning of human enhancement

Coffee in the Great Library of Alexandria

Winston: Gosh! Where on Earth are we now?

Olen: Winston, well, we aren't really "on Earth." I wonder if you remember that we made our way back to the Filthy Spoon. Physically that's where we all are, seated at our traditional table. As we all sat down I activated the neural implants that you all agreed to insert.

Eugenie: Actually, I don't remember that ...

Olen: (*Olen's avatar takes out his notepad and starts furiously typing*) OK ... (*mutters to himself*) short-term memory loss ... (*to the group*) obviously we're still working on the tech. But look where the neural lace has enabled us to have coffee.

Winston: The coffee at the Filthy Spoon was pretty bad. So what artificial reality have you created for us in the Metaverse? Will the coffee be any better?

Olen: Since we're going to be addressing the issue of what it means to be enhanced the best place to have that discussion is in a place with lots of books. So here we are at the Great Library of Alexandria.

Text appears, floating between the avatars of the friends.

The Great Library of Alexandria in Alexandria, Egypt, was one of the largest and most significant libraries of the ancient

DOI: 10.4324/9781003321613-2

world. The Library was part of a larger research institution called the Mouseion, which was dedicated to the Muses, the nine goddesses of the arts. The idea of a universal library in Alexandria may have been proposed by Demetrius of Phalerum, an exiled Athenian statesman living in Alexandria, to Ptolemy I Soter, who may have established plans for the Library, but the Library itself was probably not built until the reign of his son Ptolemy II Philadelphus. The Library quickly acquired many papyrus scrolls, owing largely to the Ptolemaic kings' aggressive and well-funded policies for procuring texts. It is unknown precisely how many such scrolls were housed at any given time, but estimates range from 40,000 to 400,000 at its height.

Alexandria came to be regarded as the capitol of knowledge and learning, in part because of the Great Library. (Library of Alexandria – Wikipedia https://en.wikipedia.org/wiki/Library_of_Alexandria)

Olen: We now have ready access to all of the wisdom in the Great Library. Just speak the name of a book and a fully searchable interface will appear.

Winston: I imagine that philosophers have had quite a lot to say about enhancement since the ancient philosopher sages whose work found its way into the Great Library. Have you updated these shelves to reflect that?

Olen: Of course! If it's anywhere on the internet, it's here.

Winston: I'm pretty confident that scholars in the Great Library weren't sipping coffee. The brews that have just appeared before us certainly taste better than the offerings of the Filthy Spoon. Are we really drinking Filthy Spoon coffee?

Olen: Sure, remember we had to keep buying bad coffee to avoid being kicked out. The bad news is that you are still drinking that terrible coffee. But I've inserted sensors that will stimulate taste centres in the brain that will make this coffee taste like the best coffee you've ever had. But there's more to this than me showing off some amazing digital tech. I have a philosophical agenda. Some of the digital technologies so magnificently on display here are easily applied to our human natures. I want you all to open your minds to the potential benefits of digital tech enhancement.

Sophie: OK, enough showing off for now, Olen! Let's all browse these virtual shelves for definitions of human enhancement.

Olen: It's all easily searchable. Everyone get busy. (*Claps hands*) Let's meet back here for coffee soon.

The friends depart to browse the Great Library's index but soon return.

Eugenie: That was a lot to take in. I'm amazed with myself how many of these abstract philosophical theories I've managed to retain.

Olen: Perhaps it's time for me to disclose something else. Effortless access to the Metaverse isn't the only benefit from your neuroprostheses. The chips have greatly enhanced your powers of memory. Last night we were told that deleting CCR5 may have given Lulu and Nana better memories. I'm betting that the digital tech cognitive boost I just gave you all was so much better than anything a gene edit gave Lulu and Nana.

Sophie: Weren't you supposed to disclose that before we agreed to have these devices inserted into our brains?

Olen: Maybe … anyway it's too late now. And the effects are fully reversible, at least, they should be. I have a bigger point to make. Philosophers and ethicists spend far too much time moaning about progress. As one of my heroes, Meta's Mark Zuckerberg said "Move Fast and Break Things!" The general ethos in tech today is that it's better to say sorry than ask permission! So sorry guys. But one thing we know about progress is that much of the stuff that gets broken won't be missed when it is replaced by shiny new stuff. I think that applies to many of the supposedly valuable aspects of human nature that enhancement technologies will break and replace. Enjoy your cognitive upgrades!

What are enhancement technologies?

Sophie: Can we backtrack a bit here. I know that the topic of today's discussion is the definition of human enhancement. But before we get on to that can I ask a question or two about *enhancement technologies*. That sounds like it should be an important category for our philosophical investigation. To prepare for the philosophical heavy lifting of defining enhancement can we get a sense, possibly approximate, of what interventions might be included in this category? Of course, I understand that we won't have a full and final definition of enhancement technologies until we have a better sense of what "enhancement" means.

Olen: I'll start! This is the most exciting time to be alive. We are now entering an *Age of Human Enhancement*. The Enlightenment gave us the scientific method which enabled a host of inventions that improved human lives. With this next stage in the Enlightenment we are turning technologies inward at our very natures. Advances in gene editing enable experimentation with DNA influencing many human traits. Nootropics, drugs that enhance cognitive functions have come to the Amazon Marketplace. He Jiankui's editing of Lulu and Nana's genomes suggests the potential for enhancement from editing the human genome. There are experiments in cybernetic brain implants and replacements for human body parts.

Sophie: So human enhancement technologies are defined by their effects on human beings? Olen, you have quickly rattled off a few examples. They seem quite varied to me. Gene edits can alter DNA. Nootropics are supposed to alter our brain chemistry. Cybernetic interventions introduce digital technologies into our brains or bodies. I'd like us to consider whether enhancement technologies are what philosophers would describe as a natural kind?

Eugenie: Sophie, can you tell us what you mean by "natural kind"?

Sophie: Plato offered a wonderful metaphor that today's philosophers use to explain a natural kind. The best theories, according to Plato, "carve nature at its joints." Plato thought that nature came predivided in ways that it was our job to discover. Our scientific theories should aim to carve nature at its joints by identifying natural kinds. Put more clumsily – and less poetically – natural kinds separate nature into objective samenesses and differences. Oxygen atoms form a natural kind because each oxygen atom is objectively similar to each other oxygen atom. They don't share these specific similarities with carbon atoms, for example.

Eugenie: I think I follow that. How are you applying this to technologies that we may use to enhance ourselves?

Sophie: I introduce the idea of natural kinds to make the point that enhancement technologies *don't* seem to be a natural kind. Rather they are a broad collection of technologies that improve some human trait that we value. But that doesn't excuse us from clarifying what to include in the category of "enhancement technology." If we name some clear cases of enhancement technologies then perhaps we can get a sense of what they share. We know that they include pharmaceutical interventions. Nootropics, drugs that enhance cognitive functions, are available for purchase in the Amazon Marketplace.

Olen: Yes, some of these are really cool. Here's one example that I take from the Amazon Marketplace. (*Olen performs a gesture and text and images from the Amazon*

Marketplace appear before the friends. There he locates "Smart Drugs." Olen gestures, apparently at random, toward a link.)

Panax ginseng root "has been shown to reduce brain fatigue and significantly improve performance on difficult tasks like mental math problems."

I'm not saying that all of these nootropics work as advertised, but there are serious scientific studies supporting claims about some smart drugs.

Eugenie: Can you offer an example that's less herbal?

Olen: OK Eugenie, I understand your scepticism. How about Modafinil. It's a pharmaceutical used to treat narcolepsy. There are studies that support the enhancing effects of Modafinil on concentration. It seems to enhance powers of attention and focus, leading some students studying for exams and poker players competing in multiday events to take it. One commentator calls Modafinil "the world's first safe smart drug."

Winston: I can see that if you plan to sign up for a multiday poker tournament then it may be a good idea to take a drug that combats the exhaustion when, by day three, all the cards you have been dealt become a fatiguing blur. But we need to consider the downsides of Modafinil. I've just located a 2009 discussion of neuroenhancers in the *New Yorker* by Margaret Talbot. She interviews Martha Farah a psychologist who conducted studies of Modafinil's cognitive effects. Farah expresses the concern that the enhancement of powers of concentration might come with a negative effect on the powers of creativity of those who take it. I like this quote from Farah "I'm a little concerned that we could be raising a generation of very focussed accountants." That kind of focus may be great, especially if you're an accountant, but what if you're a poet?

Olen: Nootropics are only the beginning. Please follow me deeper into the rabbit hole of human enhancement tech. We've already seen some speculation about gene editing as an enhancement technology. Recent advances in gene editing combine brilliantly with genomics, the study of genomes. Human genomics describes genes and how they interact to produce our cognitive and physical traits. What genomics describes genetic edits can change. We've already discussed editing CCR5. With progress in genomics and expected advances in gene editing there's so much more to come.

Sophie: So we can add gene editing and genomics to the category of enhancement technologies.

Olen: But wait, there's more! Please follow me still deeper into the enhancement rabbit hole. There are also cybernetic interventions in human cognitive or physical abilities. These digital techs should be included among enhancement technologies.

Sophie: Can you give an example of that?

Olen: Sure! You're wearing one.

Winston: (*Winston's avatar aggressively pouts.*) I'm still annoyed at that!

Sophie: How about an example that scientists have studied?

Olen: We are in the early stages of this most exciting category of enhancement technology. But one promising line of research is on hippocampal prostheses. The hippocampus is a part of the brain that, among other functions, helps in the storage and retrieval of memories. It is a part of the brain that can suffer damage in Alzheimer's disease. There is promising work on rats and monkeys to build a neuroprosthesis capable of replacing damaged hippocampi.

Winston: Somehow it's not surprising to me that this line of research will proceed by way of the suffering of nonhuman mammals. It's all for us, but they suffer.

Sophie: You raise an important issue Winston. But I suppose we're here to address the implications of this research

	for human candidates for enhancement. Please go on Olen.
Olen:	Thank you Sophie. A goal of this research is biomimicry. When introduced into a brain the hippocampal neuroprosthesis will ideally perform all the functions of the biological material it replaces.
Sophie:	So far you've been describing the early stages of what could be a promising line of research on a treatment for Alzheimer's. Can you clarify its relevance to the debate about human enhancement?
Olen:	The key point is that the hippocampal prosthesis is a digital technology. I think this will be a topic for discussion on a later evening. But effectively digital technologies get better. Suppose you design a hippocampal prosthesis that does everything that a healthy human hippocampus does. Introducing that into the brain of a patient with Alzheimer's gives them normal human capacities of memory. But it's a digital technology and will become more powerful. Today's fix for an impaired memory should give rise to a device tomorrow that grants superhuman memories. You'll be happy to hear that the ease with which you retain memories of your readings in the Great Library suggests that the neuroprostheses you are now wearing have upgraded your hippocampi.
Winston:	I'm still angry that you took it upon yourself to do that to us! Did we consent?
Olen:	Hmm … well given that you're complaining about short-term memory loss, how do you know that you didn't?
Sophie:	We now have some sense of the category of technological interventions we are talking about. I can see that these enhancement technologies differ in so many ways. They aren't a natural kind. They aren't objectively similar. Rather they all improve a trait of human beings that we value. The looseness of the category leaves open the possibility that some future genius might invent a

	quantum enhancement technology that we could add to the category of enhancement technologies.
Olen:	Yes. Thanks Sophie, I for one am really looking forward to that quantum enhancement technology!
Winston:	Enough of your tech rhapsodizing for now, Olen! Time to do some serious philosophical work. Tell us, what does it mean to enhance a human being?

What does it mean to be enhanced?

Eugenie: Let me go first. Philosophers are sometimes inclined to overcomplicate things. In this case there is a very simple definition. (*Eugenie gestures at the English dictionary section of the Library.*) To enhance is to improve. I recently enhanced my smartphone by adding memory to it. It's now better – its store of photos is boosted. Simple! You enhance a human when you do what I did to my smartphone. CCR5 deletion may have enhanced the twins' cognitive abilities simply by improving them. Now Olen, with that issue settled, can we add anything alcoholic to these virtual coffees?

Sophie: Not so fast, Eugenie. But Olen, I do want to get back to the effects of the virtual alcohol in this café's special coffees later. Eugenie, I think there are cases of human enhancement that fit your definition very well. You all know that I'm a keen runner. Enhancement *as improvement* seems to describe what I do when I train for an event. I enhance my capacity to run by exercising. There are various brain-training activities that I do on my smartphone. Perhaps these cognitively enhance me by improving my powers of concentration. They may make me a better player of contract bridge. But there are cases that challenge that definition. These cases show that we can't straightforwardly move from the suggestion that since enhancement is improvement, and improvement is, by definition, good, then enhancement is necessarily good.

Eugenie: (*yawns*) Go on, Sophie. Please display your philosophical acumen by talking us through some of these counterexamples.

Sophie: Thank you Eugenie. I want to do better than just introducing a counterexample. Let's spend a bit of time to see how disagreements about how to define human enhancement really play out in a debate that becomes big news every four years. This is the debate about performance-enhancing drugs in sport. Every four years the world's focus fixates on the summer Olympics. There are inevitably stories of athletes banned from competition or stripped of medals because they've been caught cheating. The cheating here is enhancement.

Did Ben Johnson really cheat at the 1988 Seoul Olympics?

Sophie: We are all old enough to remember when the Canadian sprinter Ben Johnson won the gold medal in the 100-metre sprint event at the 1988 Seoul Olympics in a time of 9.79 seconds. He was shown to have achieved that time with the anabolic steroid Stanozolol. Johnson was stripped of his medal. The straightforward identification of human enhancement with human improvement clearly omits details that would justify condemning Johnson. We need a better definition of human enhancement if we are to understand how Johnson's method of improving himself was wrong.

Eugenie: Not so fast, Sophie! I wonder if you are expecting too much of my simple definition. Perhaps you didn't like Johnson's method of enhancement. But it seems as straightforward a case of enhancement as improvement as the lesser results that I get from my evening jogs. My method of enhancement didn't break any rules of competition. But Johnson's did. Furthermore, I challenge the contention that there is anything really wrong in what Johnson did. I remember the thrill of watching his Seoul performance. I understand that attention to the letter of the rules of Olympic competition makes it clear that Johnson cheated. But that doesn't mean that those rules were philosophically justified.

Sophie: Go on.

Eugenie: We can all think of immoral laws – laws prohibiting homosexuality, for example. Gay people break that law but certainly don't break any law of morality. The same applies to the rule of Olympic competition that Johnson broke. Their advocates make the point that performance-enhancing drugs may be excellent expressions of the Olympic ideal. They tell the story of the historical event that inspired the marathon – the messenger Feidipides who dropped dead of exhaustion after running back to Athens to report victory over the Persian army at the Battle of Marathon in 490 BCE. I'm sure Feidipides would have appreciated any safe enhancers the Athenian generals could offer him. Johnson didn't cross the finish line in Seoul first by sabotaging his competitors. He did so by trying to run 100 metres as quickly as he possibly could. His 9.79 seconds were the purest expression of the Olympic ideal. Johnson surely knew that injecting anabolic steroids was against the rules of Olympic sport as codified now. But let's look forward to a future Olympics in which archaic rules no longer prevent humans from occasionally thrilling crowds by offering superhuman performances.

Winston: I strongly disagree with you, Eugenie! I agree that watching that Seoul final was thrilling. But I have to confess my profound sense of disappointment when it was revealed that Johnson had doped. His 9.79 seconds seemed to me to be a lie. I identify as a bioconservative opponent of human enhancement. I have no complaints whatsoever about Sophie's exercise programme. I applaud it. But Johnson's method of improvement by performance enhancing drugs was objectionable and should be condemned.

Eugenie: How was Johnson's Seoul sprint a lie? I didn't notice him getting into a car to cover that distance.

Winston: I watched that final with the belief that Johnson was competing under the conditions that govern my very human attempts to sprint 100 metres. I assure you that I don't inject Stanozolol to prepare for my morning jogs. Eugenie – you are right that Johnson didn't cover that distance in a car. But I don't see such a big difference between that and Johnson's method.

Eugenie: But Winston, there are so many things that elite athletes do that you don't to prepare for your evening jogs. I'm sorry but I'm not going to be taking time out of my busy schedule to watch you stumble 100 metres in a very human way.

Who – or what – is the world's best chess player?

Winston: I certainly have an interest in elite performance, but in elite *human* performance. I'm fascinated to see what can be achieved by someone who's basically a better version of me. We overlook the extent to which the Olympics are performances for audiences of humans. Let me clarify this with another example – chess.

Olen: Excellent, my equal favourite sport!

Winston: Ever since IBM's Deep Blue beat the then world's best chess player Garry Kasparov in 1997 it's been apparent that the planet's best chess players are no longer human. What interests me is the way we continue to be interested in the exploits of human chess players. The best chess player on the planet is no longer human but we don't seem to care that much. We follow the exploits of objectively inferior human chess players. When the best human players play against computers, it's typically to prepare for games against other humans. Deep Blue's victory over Kasparov was a world first so of course it got media attention. I don't think people are much interested in watching today's chess computers even if we know they are objectively superior to Deep Blue. No one wants to watch the best human middle-distance runners be easily beaten by someone in their Toyota Corolla sedan. There is little interest in watching chess computers duke it out against each other. Chess matches are performances for human audiences. We enjoy watching chess matches between humans just as we enjoy watching humans perform *Hamlet*. Who would pay money to watch a performance by Robo-Ophelia?

Eugenie: That sounds very clever, Winston, but doesn't it run into a philosophical obstacle? I just told you that I really enjoyed watching Johnson's performance. Are you trying to tell me I'm not human? And if I remember correctly you said you enjoyed it too until someone spoiled it by revealing the positive doping result. I'm sorry but I think there is a big difference between doping Johnson and Robo-Ophelia even if we accept your wider point that Olympic athletes are, in essence, performers for human audiences. Perhaps Johnson is a cheat but he's definitely human.

Winston: I'm not surprised you disagree with me.

Eugenie: To demonstrate my point I'm going to put a YouTube clip of Johnson's Seoul performance up here. I will run it alongside a clip of my uncle Bert driving his 2005 Corolla at maximum speed over the same distance. (*Eugenie performs the gestures to display Johnson's and Bert's performances. Everyone's eyes are fixed on Johnson. No one watches Bert in his Corolla.*)

Winston: I take your point, Eugenie. But the point I'm making is more subtle than that. The interest we have in human performances comes by degree. I'm suggesting that our interest in elite athletic performance is not 1 or 0, on or off. I think it's useful to place candidates for human performances on a spectrum. At one extreme are straightforwardly nonhuman performances. Driverless cars are manufactured by humans. But when a driverless car lacking a human assistant sets out to cover 100 metres it does so in an entirely nonhuman way. It doesn't even have Bert at the steering wheel! On a spectrum that measures humanness it scores a 0. When I jog 100 metres I score a 1 – I cover that distance in a paradigmatically human way. We've already established that my distinctively human performance is unlikely to interest many of the people who eagerly tuned in to watch Usain Bolt's record-breaking sprints. But both my and Bolt's athletic achievements are equally human. These endpoints of the athletic humanness spectrum are easily evaluated. The midpoints are less easily identified. Do you remember the late 1970s show The *Six Million Dollar Man*? Steve Austin was rebuilt with robotic parts. He's still mostly human. But with his robotic limbs his athletic performances are recognizably less human than mine or Bolt's. I conjecture that human audiences have less of an interest in Steve Austin's 100-metre sprints. Watching him compete at the Olympics would be a bit like watching mostly robotic Ophelia in *Hamlet*. Perhaps it's a bit of a leap but I think that the value of humanness explains my sense of betrayal about Johnson's Seoul performance. Johnson is assuredly human. But his 9.79 seconds was less human than it purported to be.

Eugenie: But still thrilling and exceptional! Sorry Winston but I wasn't really listening to you. There's a rewind feature that let me rewatch Johnson's sprint, editing Bert out. It's a truly riveting *human* performance.

Winston: To clarify my interest as a human spectator, I watched that final with the belief that Johnson's performance was telling me something about what might have been possible for me had I been a bit more talented and athletically committed. To put this value of athletic humanness in terms that money-oriented Olen might understand, I'd pay less to see doping athletes compete than I would to see clean human athletes run the same distance slightly slower.

Eugenie: (*Eugenie's avatar seems to be getting grumpy*) I'm still not getting it! I saw you watching that YouTube replay of Johnson's Seoul performance. I don't think you glanced once at poor uncle Bert in his Corolla.

Winston: Perhaps the point is easier to grasp at the extremes and with the intellectual sport of chess. I would pay a lot to watch the current world chess champion Magnus Carlsen play. But I wouldn't pay anything to be present while two of Olen's computers running different chess programs competed even though I fully understand that Carlsen's chess play is objectively inferior. I'd watch once for the novelty. But then I'd do something else. I'm not a great chess player, but the thrill for me in watching him is wondering what's going on in his head as he ponders his next move. Watching back over Carlsen's games I really enjoy observing his moves and imaginatively putting myself in his position at the chess board. I'm inspired to think through the reasoning that he went through as he prepared to make that daring queen sacrifice. I don't feel at all tempted to ponder what's going on in the head of Olen's chess computer. Would it be a long stream of 0s and 1s? It reminds me of the binary solo that concludes the New Zealand comedy duo *Flight of the Conchords'* song "The Humans are Dead." (*Winston plays the final verses of that song.*) Here are some lines sung by robots celebrating the demise of humanity.

Binary solo!
0000001
00000011
000000111
00001111

Perhaps these 0s and 1s are thrilling for robots, but not so good for humans.

Olen: Thanks for your entirely expected ill will, Winston. But I think you've refuted yourself by playing that *Flight of the Conchords* clip. I loved it. Chess machines are fascinating to observe and to struggle to understand. I'm not sure if you've kept up with the revolutions in play that brought the AlphaGo program of DeepMind Technologies. DeepMind is a subsidiary of Google. Its approach to strategy games like chess and Go make IBM's Deep Blue program look positively antiquated. By the way, Go is my equal favourite sport with chess.

Eugenie: Yes, I figured chess wouldn't be equal favourite with rugby!

Winston: I can see I will never convince you, Olen. We may have to agree to differ. But I will say that fascinating though the story of AlphaGo is, I find it interesting mainly as an oddity. I watched and loved the 2017 Netflix documentary *AlphaGo*. It covered DeepMind's unexpected defeat of the Korean Go champion Lee Sedol. Sedol went into that match confident that no computer could beat him and received his comeuppance. The story of DeepMind was amazing. But for me the star of that movie was the chain-smoking Lee Sedol as he bore the hopes and expectations of all of Go-playing humanity. I was so disappointed to read of Sedol's retirement from the game, seemingly triggered by his defeat by AlphaGo. Sedol said "Even if I become the number one, there is an entity that cannot be defeated." I wanted to say "Please Lee, continue playing. Play for us." I'm a rubbish Go player but I'd definitely pay to watch you play. I couldn't care less about what AlphaGo goes on to do after its defeat of Sedol. After its victory over Kasparov, Deep Blue is now a museum exhibit in the Smithsonian National Museum of American History. I don't think people are wondering much about what it would have been thinking or doing if IBM hadn't switched it off.

Olen: Thanks for clarifying your commitment to human mediocrity, Winston.

Winston: Thanks Olen. But I'm interested in elite performance within or just beyond human norms. That account of enhancement that explains my lack of interest in the objectively superior performances of AlphaGo and Johnson on Stanozolol. I'm a committed fan of the British premier league team Burnley. I watch the exceptional efforts of their players even if I know that pressing a button on my remote will take me to the objectively superior play of Manchester City. I think my human commitment to exceptional performances within human limits is a bit like my commitment to Burnley. I'm disappointed when they lose to a clearly superior team but I retain my interest much in the way I'd love to see the objectively inferior Sedol play Go. I'm interested in Sedol's performances because I'm human. I figure that if I were an extraterrestrial or future artificial intelligence I wouldn't care so much.

Sophie: I've enjoyed listening to this exchange. I've noticed my credences – degrees of belief – shifting with each new line of argument. So thank you! Ben Johnson knew, or should have known, that he was breaking the rules of Olympic competition. But isn't that more a moral indictment of the rules than of the athlete? To tell you the truth I don't know what to think about doping in sport right now. One thing that might help is translating these thoughts about performance-enhancing drugs in sport into a new definition of enhancement. Eugenie's original definition – enhancement as improvement – seems to endorse Johnson's doping. Winston, do you have any thoughts about a definition of enhancement that would support your condemnation of Johnson?

Winston: I am sceptical about using tech to enhance humans. But I'm certainly in favour of people committing to exercise programmes or seeking to make themselves mentally sharper by playing lots of Sudoku. I do think these efforts differ from the variety of technologies that Olen seems so excited about directing at our human natures.

Eugenie: Sorry Winston, we're going to need more than some vague suspicions.

Winston: Here's something I offer as a working definition. It will sound vague to begin with, especially compared with Eugenie's philosophically straightforward identification of human enhancement with human improvement. But I think this is a point in its favour. The enhancement technologies that Olen has described potentially affect so many human values. I quote Albert Einstein's observation that "Everything should be made as simple as possible, but not simpler." Philosophers have spent millennia debating and clarifying human values so it's no surprise that it won't be easy to precisely define how enhancement technologies affect these values. I'm going to venture a definition in the expectation that it will be clarified through your criticism.

Olen: (*eagerly rubbing his hands*) So you're offering a definition with the expectation that we will be able to demolish it. This should be fun!

Winston: OK. Here's a first pass at a definition that begins with a distinction between two kinds of human improvement. One purpose of intervening in human capacities is therapy. If you have a sore throat resulting from a bacterial infection you might take an antibiotic. If the antibiotic clears the bacteria it restores your throat to normal health. Therapeutic improvement – the restoration of biologically normal levels of functioning – is the goal of medicine. I'm going to exclude these interventions from the category of human enhancement. Enhancements will be technological interventions that aim to improve human function beyond biologically normal levels. This is what distinguishes them from therapeutic tech interventions.

Sophie: I see that you have made specific reference to technology here. There's therefore a connection with the category of enhancement technologies. I'm a philosopher used to operating at the level of pure principle. But I think I need an example or two. Olen identifies human enhancements with human improvements. This explains his endorsement of technological enhancement. If to enhance is to make better, then it follows that it must be good. I can see that. Now Winston is subdividing human improvements into therapies and enhancements. He's telling us that the therapeutic uses of technology are good.

Winston: Yes, that's right. But there's more to say about uses of technology to enhance. I'm not saying that they are all bad. I'm saying that they are all *morally problematic.*

Olen: (*Olen's avatar looks frustrated*) I certainly need some philosophical clarity on this! Winston, are you actually saying anything? Morally problematic?! This sounds like another way to say morally wrong. Would you do us the courtesy of saying what you mean. Sophie, can you insist that Winston say what he means?

Winston: By morally problematic I mean only that it raises a moral problem. Whether it's morally or prudentially good will depend on what other values it might conflict with. I'm informed here by my reading of the many varied reflections on what it means to be human in the Great Library. I'm pleased that the Library includes philosophical reflections that go beyond the Western intellectual tradition. I'm beginning to suspect that the use of technological means to improve beyond human norms may conflict with other important values. But I'm still thinking about what these might be. For the time being I want to label these interventions as morally problematic. Olen turned us all into guinea pigs when he implanted these neuroprostheses in our brain. (*Winston shakes a virtual fist at Olen.*) But now that we have them, let's do our best to take in as many different perspectives as possible on what it means to be human and what's valuable about remaining so.

The morally problematic nature of Sophie's insulin pump

Sophie: I think I follow you. Here's an example I would like you to help me with Winston. I'm still struggling with this concept of "morally problematic." You know that I have diabetes. I am the beneficiary of some technology that compensates for my faulty pancreas. My insulin pump secretes insulin. It improves my capacity to regulate my blood sugar. But since that improvement is only up to and not beyond biologically normal levels then it's morally unproblematic, right?

Winston: One thing I really don't like about philosophers is the way you come up with objections I hadn't expected. Now I'm going to have to do some thinking aloud, on my feet. What would I say about your pump? Here's a first thought, but I am thinking on my feet, inventing this as I go along.

Sophie: I think Socrates might be impressed by your expression of epistemic modesty. Perhaps we can work together to resolve the philosophical complexities of my insulin pump. Four minds are better than one.

Winston: Well Sophie, I certainly don't want to take your pump away from you.

Sophie: Thanks Winston. But to adapt actor and NRA member Charlton Heston's defence of his right to bear arms, I'll give you my insulin pump when you pry it from my cold, dead hands!

Winston: Message received! Can I say that your pump is an application of technology to a human body and that makes it morally problematic, but only in the sense that the question should be asked. Whenever you are combining human biology and technology questions need to be asked. It would be philosophically remiss to let them pass without comment. In this case questions are fairly easily answered. And I'm not just talking about your diabetic Charlton Heston act. It's clear that your technology does for you what my pancreas does for me. Problem solved!

Sophie: Thanks Winston. I feel like I can stand down now. But I have a further question for you, not so much about this pump. (*Sophie gestures at her midriff, and looks puzzled.*) I notice that feature of me has not been replicated in my avatar. I'm not sure what I think about that. It seems that Olen's tech has given me what it takes to be a non-diseased, non-disabled version of me without bothering to ask me what I thought about that. It just assumed that in the ideal world I would choose to be non-diabetic.

Olen: Sorry Sophie. But my assumptions were based on your long history of moaning about all the irritations and inconveniencies of being diabetic.

Sophie: Actually, my question isn't about that. I'm interested in what you would say about a future improvement of my pump. In my years as a diabetic using a pump I've noticed significant improvements in the technology. Telling my pump what to do used to be an awkward process. My selection of my insulin doses involved a lot of guess work. This new pump is connected to a sensor. It applied machine learning to patterns in my need for insulin. It now chooses when and how much insulin to give me. The longer I wear it, the better it seems to know me.

Winston: Fingers crossed that this intelligent machine won't decide, like the artificial intelligence Skynet in the *Terminator* movies, that the world is a better place without Sophie.

Olen: I wouldn't worry about that, Sophie. What works as the premise for a successful Hollywood movie franchise doesn't necessarily make for a useful prediction of the future of artificial intelligence. But I don't think that's your question, is it, Sophie?

Sophie: No, it isn't. I'm wondering what you would say about upgrades of my pump that improved its functioning to levels beyond healthy biological pancreases? Over time supposedly healthy pancreases get worse at regulating blood sugar. There is a state many find themselves in as they age. They become prediabetic. They aren't diabetic, but they could be headed in that direction. The pumps of the future could outperform the pancreases of many prediabetic people. But I'm interested in possibilities beyond even that. Olen's advocacy of digital technologies suggests a future in which I might enjoy a superhuman digital pancreas. Would you condemn me in the way you seem to want to condemn Johnson? That just sounds like envy.

Winston: Good question, Sophie. I'm thinking I should say that your superhuman digital pancreas is morally problematic. But again, when I ask the question there seems little reason to condemn it. Perhaps the use of technology to take us beyond biologically normal levels is morally problematic in a way that therapeutic improvements are not. We should ask questions. But I think we should solve the problems of your potentially superhuman insulin pump in favour of your continued access to it.

Sophie: Thank you Winston. I suspect you may be tiring of all of my questions and distinctions. But I think I need to make one more.

Winston: OK Sophie, but *just one*!

Sophie: I hear you, Winston. When we ask questions about which changes to human beings are good we should distinguish *morally* good interventions from *prudentially* good interventions. Prudentially good changes to human attributes are good for the individual who receives them. There's a contrast with morally good changes which take into account the interests of others. If you think that Johnson's use of Stanozolol was immoral then it was a morally bad change. But if he had managed to get away with it you might say that it was prudentially good. Johnson will have benefited by cheating.

Eugenie: I think I follow that distinction. Of course, I disagree with your moral assessment. The way you are introducing this suggests that we should store this distinction away for future philosophical use.

Sophie: Correct! I think it will prove useful.

Moving on

Olen: OK ... I think ...Sophie, are you happy for us to move on to serious discussion of enhancement technologies with this seemingly vague and incomplete sense of what we're talking about?

Sophie: Actually, I am. Scientists often begin their explorations with working definitions of the phenomena they're talking about. Biologists' working definitions of genes sufficed to get their investigations underway. But these working definitions weren't much like the definitions that today's biologists would accept. I think our two working definitions of enhancement, together with the other distinctions we have introduced, will certainly get us underway.

Olen: If you say so.

Sophie: We've got two morally contrasting definitions. By "morally contrasting" I mean that they seem aligned to two different views about enhancement. First, we have *enhancement as improvement*. This seems to suggest endorsement of enhancing humans. Second, we have *enhancement by technological means beyond human norms*. If I understand Winston correctly, this seems to support a different evaluation. Improvements up to biological norms are endorsed. But improvements beyond human norms by technological means are problematic. They deserve further investigation and may turn out to be morally or prudentially bad depending on how they interact with other values. We've also said that we should distinguish between enhancements as morally good or bad, and between enhancements as prudentially good or bad.

Olen: I thought philosophers were supposed to offer definitions that simplified things. Does this mean that we are at least temporarily done with the philosophical navel-gazing and are ready to get on with discussing with really exciting technologies that we can soon apply to our bodies and brains?

Eugenie: Not so fast, Olen. We have some history do deal with. I can tell that, for you, enhancement is all about applying exciting new technologies to our human natures. You can't wait to tell us all about pharmaceuticals designed to sharpen us intellectually, how our genes can be edited to extend our lifespans, or how cybernetic implants can be attached to us significantly boosting out intellects. But human enhancement has a history that predates these technologies. We will need a detour through the history of eugenics.

Winston: Hear, hear, Eugenie! Your avatar has adopted an optimistic pose. But I've been doing some browsing in the Great Library, and eugenics is much more a cautionary tale than a message of hope for an enhanced future. Sorry Olen.

Olen: Boo!

Night 3 From Francis Galton's eugenics to liberal eugenics

Coffee in the offices of the Royal Geographical Society in late 1800s London

Sophie: So where are we now? And, who brought us here? Looks like we've done some time travelling!

Eugenie: I chose tonight's venue. We're in late 1800s London – more specifically in the offices of the Royal Geographical Society. It's a learned society whose purpose is the "advancement of geographical science." But don't worry – Olen assures me that the virtual coffee is just as good as at the Great Library and we retain access to its catalogue. I chose this location to explore what might be the genesis of scientific attempts to enhance humanity.

Winston: Excellent choice, Eugenie. We all badly need a history lesson or two before Olen burdens our brains with stories about millennial lifespans and flying cars.

Francis Galton and eugenics

Eugenie: If we are going to talk about human enhancement, we need to find out where the idea of using science to improve humanity came from. One of the distinguished members of the Royal Geographical Society at this time was Francis Galton, a polymath brainbox who was a cousin of Charles Darwin. He learned from cousin Charles in

DOI: 10.4324/9781003321613-3

a way that should be a lesson for us. Galton coined the term *eugenics*, a combination of the Greek *eu*, meaning "good" or "well," and *genēs*, meaning "born." Here's his definition. (*Eugenie has now mastered the Metaverse gestures that display text before them.*)

Eugenics is "the science of improving stock, which is by no means confined to questions of judicious mating, but which, especially in the case of man, takes cognizance of all influences that tend in however remote a degree to give to the more suitable races or strains of blood a better chance of prevailing speedily over the less suitable."

Winston: Thanks Eugenie. If you aren't already alarmed about this talk about more or less suitable races, Galton was a terrible racist. Here's a letter he wrote in 1873 to the *Times* of London, "Africa for the Chinese," in which he suggested that the world would be better off if the Chinese, "a race capable of high civilization," were to displace African people in Africa. You definitely don't want to trust someone like him to choose what kinds of people are allowed to exist. I agree with Eugenie that before we get too excited about enhancement technologies, we must learn from history. But I think she and I are going to strongly disagree about the lessons we should learn.

Eugenie: I don't want to defend any of Galton's racism. But can I at least say that Galton was a Victorian Englishman and not free of the prejudices of his age? His cousin Charles said some pretty morally objectionable things too, but we still celebrate him as the founder of evolutionary theory. Thanks to Olen's cognitively enhancing neuroprostheses, I've been doing a lot of reading and I've decided that eugenics can be defended if we tidy it up a bit. The version I would defend is "liberal eugenics." This is a view advanced by New Zealand philosopher Nicholas Agar in a 2004 book *Liberal Eugenics*.

Winston: A New Zealander? Aren't they all about rugby? Before you recklessly advance this new-fangled *liberal* eugenics, I do hope that your reading informed you about some of the horrors perpetrated in the name of eugenics.

Sophie: Yes Eugenie, not to join a pile on, but I always thought of eugenics as one of those terrible moral offences of the Nazis. Doesn't it belong in the same moral universe as the Holocaust? Can you update me Eugenie? I prepared for this discussion by watching a very informative documentary on the Nazi's T4 euthanasia programme in which disabled people were murdered in the interests of the betterment of the race. The idea was these disabled people were manifestly "bad in birth." If they were allowed to survive their poor-quality hereditary material would be passed on to the next generation. According to the documentary, between 275,000 and 300,000 disabled people were murdered. I also learned that eugenic programmes weren't limited to the Nazis. The Holocaust was a moral offence specific to the Nazis, but eugenics wasn't. Eugenic programmes were instituted before World War II across Europe, North America, and Australasia. The Nazis went further with eugenics. But in other nations there were sterilizations and legal sanctions to prevent the supposedly dysgenic from reproducing. I'm wondering what about this could serve as a guide to humanity's plans to technologically improve itself.

Eugenie: Time to cite Godwin's Law, the idea that the longer a discussion on the internet goes the closer the probability of comparisons to the Nazis or Adolf Hitler gets to 1. Yes, the Nazis were morally vile. But it's silly to reject an idea just because some evil people also liked it. I support public health campaigns to reduce smoking rates even if these were pioneered in Nazi Germany. Hitler was an avowed non-smoker. It's clear that Galton held some morally abhorrent views, but I'm glad Winston agrees that it's best to begin our exploration of enhancement with eugenics.

Winston: Thanks Eugenie. Except what I am nominating as a warning from history you are choosing to advocate? (*Winston's avatar adopts a horrified expression.*) It's important that we not minimize the lessons from history. We must understand that eugenic attitudes are still present and its effects are still felt by the disabled and other marginalized people.

Sophie: Perhaps we need to learn about some of Galton's ideas before we decide if any of them can help.

Eugenie: Thanks Sophie. Galton makes a distinction between *negative* eugenics which was supposed to involve preventing the genetically unfortunate from reproducing, and *positive* eugenics which was about encouraging the genetically fortunate to reproduce. Galton was confident that this would lead to an enhanced humanity because it was essentially the method of selective breeding that farmers had successfully used to improve the quality of their livestock. Selective planting and breeding provided the nutritious and nourishing meals that powered humanity's ascent to civilization. So why not try it on us? Given time, the selective breeding of humans should accelerate the processes of evolutionary improvement eventually producing smarter, healthier, longer-lived humans.

The ethical fix of "liberal" eugenics

Sophie: Sorry to confirm Godwin's Law, but is the complaint about the Nazis not that they were eugenicists, but that they were rejected some of the moral safeguards that ethical eugenicists should observe?

Eugenie: Humans are not livestock! It would be deeply immoral to seek to enhance humanity by managing human reproduction. The version of eugenics I would defend is liberal. I'm a liberal who strongly supports the idea of individuals having the right to make important choices about their lives. Toward the top of that list of important liberties are procreative freedoms, individuals' rights to choose whether they have children at all, when then have children, with whom they have children, how many children they have. A woman's right to terminate a pregnancy is part of this broader liberty.

Sophie: So how does this make your liberal view different from Galton's eugenics?

Eugenie: Galton's eugenics was authoritarian. It did not respect procreative liberty. Liberal eugenicists respect and extend it. They offer, as a novel addition to the scope of procreative freedom, the liberty to choose some of your children's hereditary material.

Sophie: So authoritarian eugenicists argue against procreative freedom, whereas liberal eugenicists significantly extend it?

Eugenie: That's right, Sophie. In this view, negative eugenics becomes the most offensive trespass on procreative freedom. It involved denying people the right to have children on the grounds that their hereditary material might lead to a decline in the quality of a given population. Positive eugenics isn't particularly positive when viewed from a moral standpoint. It involves directions to reproduce. The supposedly hereditarily fortunate were subject to a moral obligation to have children. Not passing on their high-quality hereditary material would be a moral offence. People should be morally empowered to be childless regardless of some expert's assessment of their inborn qualities. We should be deeply suspicious about anyone who claims to be an expert about what kinds of people should be allowed to exist.

Winston: Can you hear yourself, Eugenie? This all sounds terrible. Surely you can't believe that adding the epithet "liberal" can turn this moral atrocity into a something good? What's next, Nice Nazism?

Eugenie: Enough with your Nazi references, Winston. I think "liberal" is precisely the fix that eugenics needs. And that's basically because it turns decisions about enhancement over to individuals. Under authoritarian eugenics the state, informed by the relevant scientific experts, would manage reproduction, choosing who gets to reproduce much in the way a farmer scrutinizes her livestock and decides which animals to breed from. The farmer wouldn't think of asking her prize heifers whether they *want* to reproduce or asking whether a bull might actually prefer life as a sterile steer. Under liberal eugenics the state hands those decisions over to individuals. This transforms eugenics from the abnegation of procreative freedom into a doctrine that dramatically extends and enhances the reach and power of procreative choice. Prospective parents will be empowered by the new knowledge of human heredity from genomics. They will use this knowledge to guide how they use gene-editing tools to select some of their children's characteristics.

Winston: Eugenie, your affirmation of liberal eugenics strikes me as highly suspect. But before that, I have a question for Olen about this delicious coffee. If I add a shot of Drambuie to my coffee then will I get drunk?

Olen: Do you want to?

Winston: It might make this discussion more fun. I'm trying to clarify in my mind precisely how Eugenie's retread of eugenics is really an improvement on Galtonian or Nazi eugenics, so I do feel like a drink or two. But I do have work tomorrow. There are so many committees that, as a new academic, I'm expected to serve on.

Olen: Sure! This is a prototype but hangover-free drunkenness should be doable.

Winston: I'll go for the hangover free special coffee. (*He takes a few sips.*) Hmm. That is nice, and warming, and inspires me to ask my question with an appropriate emotional aspect.

   (*shouting*) Eugenie – you must be joking! Do you know how powerful and corrosive a force racism is in our society? Have you considered the possibility of morally misguided parents editing their children's genomes to reinforce their whiteness? Even worse, what about non-white parents looking around at the economic advantages that come from whiteness and, much though it pains them, modifying their children's genomes to more closely approximate the economically dominant phenotype. Sophie, you're the philosopher here. Can you call out this philosophically fraudulent malarkey?

Eugenie: Whoa there, Winston! Let's not get too carried away.

Sophie: One thing I've learned in philosophy is to not give too much weight to expressions of emotion. Winston, it's great that you're enjoying your hangover-free special coffee, but can you express your point with less vehemence and find an example that we can discuss. One of philosophy's most important tools is the philosophical thought experiment involving a counterexample. The counterexample could involve an actual case or it could be imaginary. If the case you describe is imaginary it must be consistent with known laws of logic and physics. But within those constraints you can give free rein to your imagination.

Eugenie: Thanks Sophie, but I'm worried that encouraging philosophers to give "free rein" to their imaginations may just encourage then to come up with nonsense.

Sophie: I guess that's a risk. And it would play into popular prejudices about philosophy. But it's a risk we should accept here. We are talking about the future of applying powerful enhancement technologies to our natures. In Galton's day would-be enhancers may have been limited to selective breeding. But as we saw last night, we should expect any conclusions about eugenics that we arrive at to apply to a wide range of increasingly powerful enhancement technologies. We should at least ask ourselves what Galton might done had we supplied him with twenty-first century genomics and gene editing. I'm seeking thought experiments that test the moral limits of liberal eugenics. I insist only that the counterexamples involve applications of enhancement technologies to our natures that are logically possible and are consistent with our understanding of the laws of nature.

Olen: So no stories about editing time travel genes into human genomes? They do sound fun. But I accept that restriction.

Sophie: The requirement for stories to comply with the laws of nature will ban other logically possible human enhancements. Many of the enhanced beings of fiction can fly. I'm thinking of the morally excellent Superman and his evil counterpart Homelander in the Amazon series *The Boys*. We can easily imagine them leaping into the air and flying faster than a speeding bullet but I doubt that the laws of nature would permit beings who look like them to do anything like that.

Olen: Disappointing. But this does nevertheless leave a lot of territory for imaginative exploration.

A thought experiment involving an enhanced Himmler

Winston: OK, since we've already confirmed Godwin's Law about this case, Eugenie, you want to turn eugenic choices over to parents. Suppose you have a couple who are convinced white supremacist Nazis. They have a clear sense of the kind of child they'd most like. They know how they would like to apply genomic and gene-editing technologies to the genome of their future child.

Eugenie: Are you cribbing from the plot of the 1970s movie *The Boys from Brazil?* in which evil scientists clone Hitler?

Winston: Actually, I'm imagining something much worse. This is a thought experiment remember. And also the choices of our white supremacist parents don't depend on cloning the Fuhrer and hoping for the best. Even Hitler's genome probably included elements recognized as dysgenic by Nazi race scientists. In this thought experiment

Nazi geneticists have identified genes linked with psychological traits that would empower the ruthless eradication of peoples assessed as inferior, ignoring their pleas for mercy. Even the most objectionable Nazis could have been improved upon, from this perspective. The New Zealand philosopher Jonathan Bennett – yes, another Kiwi – used one of the most hideous Nazis – the leader of the SS, Reichsführer Heinrich Himmler – to illustrate the dangers of permitting moral principles that you might be persuaded by to dominate your emotions. Himmler is correctly remembered as one of the architects of the Holocaust. But it seems that he felt emotionally tormented by the choices he made. Himmler felt terrible about all the killings directed by his Nazi moral code. Himmler is an actual case. But since we are open to imaginary counterexamples how about a Himmler enhanced according to the Nazi moral code. Himmler could have more easily done what he believed to be morally right if he'd been more psychopathic. This "enhanced Himmler" would not feel misery about the murders he commands. Instead, he would feel joy at deaths directed by Nazi morality. There doesn't seem to be anything logically or physically impossible about the enhanced Himmler.

Eugenie: Enough Winston! Olen, is it possible to turn off the tap on Winston's virtual grog? Can we remember that what you've presented is just a story. We've heard that the future is impossible to precisely predict. What stops me from telling a nasty story in which white supremacists gain power over the technologies we are developing to combat climate change and using them to save only white people from the ravages of flooding and desertification. I'm not saying it would be a fun process, but I bet if you gave me time I could come up with a nightmare future scenario in which that happens. I could make it consistent with the laws of logic and physics. Does that mean that we should cease trying to invent technologies that help with climate change?

Sophie: Winston, I can see that if pushed to extremes your philosophical strategy might be used to rebut any proposal about how to make a better future. But I do think that we should pay attention to Winston's enhanced Himmler thought experiment. Eugenie, perhaps Winston will be mollified if you can present a safeguard that would prevent Winston's imagined enhanced Himmler from coming into existence. Philosophers do like telling stories about Nazis, perhaps too much. But one thing that recent history has taught, is that there are actual people who, if given the option, would make the uses of enhancement technologies that Winston's imagined racist parents make.

What is procreative liberty?

Eugenie: Thanks Sophie. That's a reasonable request. Let me start by clarifying what it means to philosophically endorse procreative liberty. I support prospective parents' rights to choose the genetic material of future children. But I do not support *all* such choices. Liberals endorse limits on the freedoms they advocate. For example, I support the freedom of speech. But I think you should be arrested if you scream "Fire!" in a crowded passenger jet when there's clearly no fire. It should be no defence that you manage to identify advocacy of some important political view with your shouted monosyllable.

Sophie: Surely all philosophers acknowledge that.

Eugenie: You'd be surprised. In his discussion of eugenics the famous German philosopher Jürgen Habermas said of the implications of the liberal view that "decisions regarding the genetic composition of children should not be submitted to any regulation by the state, but rather should be left to the parents."

That would be a terrible implication of the liberal view. But it's surely wrong. Liberal states rightly regulate many choices that we acknowledge as free. Liberal states grant parents significant latitude on how to raise their children. But they will intervene if they deem some of your parental choices to constitute abuse. The free choices of parents in liberal societies are regulated by the state even if Habermas says they aren't.

Sophie: Habermas? Luckily, we've still got access to this fully updated Great Library of Alexandria.

Eugenie: I was hoping to not give these ideas undeserved publicity. Habermas may be Germany's most famous current philosopher and social theorist, but his arguments in that work are a bit of an embarrassment.

Winston: That hasty dismissal makes me curious. Can we take a break so I can acquaint myself with Habermas's work? I suspect that I might like a view that provokes such anger in you Eugenie.

Olen: This history of scientifically misguided ideas about enhancing humanity is depressing. I suggest that while Winston peruses Habermas the rest of us get busy with some of this fine hangover-free Shiraz virtually sourced from South Australia's Barossa Valley.

Winston seats himself in a comfy chair and the rest head to the bar.

Sophie: OK Eugenie. So how are we to prevent supposedly free prospective parents in the grip of an evil ideology from using gene editing to make morally terrible procreative choices?

Eugenie: I think the prospects are good. If two white supremacist people meet, fall in love, and decide to have children believing that their combinations of genes will produce someone even closer to the white ideal than either of them individually, then what can be done? You can't criminalize reproduction by people with obnoxious moral ideals. If racist parents choose to home-school their children the state has very little opportunity to stop them from teaching race science or a version of the history of World War II in which the real goodies lost, so long as they teach basic arithmetic and literacy.

Sophie: So you're saying that genetic selection is no worse than what already occurs?

Eugenie: Actually, I think the situation with evilly motivated genetic selection is better than what can already occur. Racist people can already consciously select their children's genes by falling in love with each other and being thrilled about a future reproductive act that will bring their child closer to the Master Race. They already can home-school their children to add what they consider the moral finishing touches.

Winston: (*getting up from his armchair*) So how would throwing enhancement technologies into this toxic mix be an improvement?

How the liberal state can prevent morally bad procreative choices

Eugenie: I've suggested that the liberal state shouldn't make our procreative choices for us. Authoritarian eugenicists supposed that there was a template for humanity. But this is not so. Liberal eugenics permits prospective parents to choose some of their children's genetic material. But we've seen that they aren't committed to anything as wide-ranging as Habermas seemed to suppose. There are limits. Just as there are expressions of the freedom of speech that should be banned, there are uses of procreative technologies that a liberal state should prohibit. The good news is that they can. I can't prevent two racist people from falling in love and having children. But suppose I am an employee of a liberal state who operates a genetic selection facility. I can and certainly should refuse to comply with their requests for assistance to

	produce a child that approximates to their obnoxious ideal.
Olen:	A benefit of the nanny state in your liberal eugenic version of the future?
Eugenie:	Sure, here's a thought experiment to clarify the role of a liberal state when faced with requests to use its tech to promote racist ends. Perhaps you can't stop the racist couple from having sex. But you can refuse any requests that you assist them. Suppose the couple resolves that lieder by Schubert would be the perfect accompaniment for their procreative efforts. You are an accomplished singer of Schubert's lieder. They approach you to accompany their procreative efforts and explain their plan. You are perfectly entitled to refuse their request for assistance. And surely you should.
Sophie:	Thinking about my mum and dad having sex always used to creep me out. But this is even worse. But how is this crazy story helping, Eugenie?
Eugenie:	I think this should describe how the agents of the liberal state should respond to requests to use genetic selection technologies. The version of liberal eugenics that I defend would insist on a state monopoly on the tools of genetic modification. The state wouldn't get to choose how you enhance your child but it would offer the same kind of moral vetting on procreative choices as it does on speech. No shouting "Fire!" on a crowded passenger jet and no selection of genetic material to bring a child closer to a racist ideal. Saying yes to that request makes me, as an agent of the state, complicit in a racist agenda. It's not illegal for citizens of a liberal state to be racist, but agents of that state must scrupulously refuse to let reproductive technologies they control be used to make a more racist society.
Sophie:	So can you tell us how, as an official of the liberal state, you would respond to a request to make racist use of enhancement technologies that you administer?

Eugenie: I would say that if you can't convince me and other members of the genetic enhancement panel that you aren't using technology that the state rightfully controls to pursue an immoral end then we say no. Today we are rightly worried about the rise of racism on the internet. The officials in a liberal state that implemented a liberal eugenics would enforce a blanket ban on attempts to alter the skin colour of future children. One of the themes of recent advances in gene editing is how much easier genetic selection is today than it was twenty years ago. I would be strongly in favour of the police in a liberal state ruthlessly cracking down on any attempt by non-state actors to control and make available tools of human genetic selection.

Sophie: Thanks Eugenie. I'm certainly not convinced, but that's helpful. But I now have another concern. Perhaps shifting decisions about how to use genetic technologies from the state to individuals makes a difference. But is this really eugenics? Isn't eugenics all about experts using their supposedly superior understanding of humanity's future to produce a society of optimal humans.

Eugenie: That's where the "liberal" helps.

Habermas responds to liberal eugenics

Sophie: Fair enough, but then let me pursue this concern from the other direction. If we're all pretending to be good liberals what about the subject of all this enhancement? The child doesn't get to choose.

Eugenie: Well, I don't see the difference between genetic interventions that shape a child's life and educational interventions. Some parents send their children to schools that educate them in accordance with the tenets of a religion. Olen, your parents sent you to a school that offered education informed by a religious ideology. I remember that, as a teenager, you seemed to know more about the commands of the Good Book than about algebra. But your successes as a tech entrepreneur show that you made up for that.

Winston: Perhaps this is a good time to reintroduce the ideas of Habermas to the debate. Reading from his book I am worried about a conflict between your supposedly liberal eugenics, Eugenie, and a deeper understanding of what it means to be a citizen in a liberal society. Here's something useful from Habermas. Unsurprisingly, I like his work more than you do, Eugenie.

According to Habermas, it's important to have origins as individuals external to the socialization process. We may have the misfortune of being socialized in a morally evil way – here I'm thinking of the example of the white supremacist parents that we keep coming back to. But at least the child had an origin that was protected from those influences. Their parents may have listened to Schubert's songs during the procreative act but that's not a proven method of selecting DNA in accordance with racist ideals.

Habermas says of the "programming intentions" of parents who seek to genetically enhance their children that they "have the peculiar status of a one-sided and unchallengeable expectation." We are familiar with the idea of children rebelling against the expectations of parents. I had a school friend who rebelled as soon has she heard the Sex Pistols' "God save the queen, The fascist regime." Sophie, your parents sent you to that elite school and gave you many social advantages. But you rebelled. I remember when you were briefly a Maoist. If your parents get to you before you were born then even that possibility is gone.

Eugenie: I'm going to respond to your Sex Pistols with some Pink Floyd – "Another Brick in the Wall." "We don't need no education, We don't need no thought control." Education *is* mind control. But it teaches is how to get by in society even as it arranges our conformity to the values of that society. Western commentators expressed surprise at the fact that so many intelligent, educated Russians endorsed Putin's invasion of Ukraine. But that's the way education and a whole bunch of other societal influences shape us and our values.

Winston: Your point??

Eugenie: Well, you've convinced me the selection of genes can be morally problematic. So following the philosopher musicians Pink Floyd, is education.

Winston: You're missing Habermas's deeper point that there isn't even the merest possibility of objecting to choices about you that occur before you're born. You are right that many acts of rebellion at evil educational influences fail. But at least they can occur.

Eugenie: I think Habermas is wrong to say that children have any realistic right of reply to the moral education that fits them to their society. But to respond to his "deeper" point, there's no huge difference between mind control by education and mind control by the selection of genes. Both influence the development of our brains.

Winston: But Habermas is correct that the selection of my genes occurs before I exist, so he's surely right to say that there is no possibility of the child having any say there.

Eugenie: I wonder. You're right that a child can't choose her own DNA. She's born with her genes. Some of the technologies that excite Olen may enable post-natal genetic self-modification. But we clearly aren't talking about those possibilities here. I nevertheless think a child can exercise control over her genes that doesn't amount to changing letters of DNA.

Winston: How so?

Eugenie: What matters is not so much the sequence of DNA that comprises your genome, rather it's the contribution that DNA makes as you grow up. There are plenty of ways in which you can influence that. It's useful to think about the example of genes that increase your cancer risk. There are no, or few, cancer genes that give you cancer from conception or birth. But there are many genetic variants that increase your probability of getting certain cancers. Inheriting a version of the gene that increases your risk of bowel cancer differs from having bowel cancer. You can make lifestyle choices that reduce your likelihood of getting cancer. Medical geneticists will say that much of the point of telling you that you've inherited a "cancer gene" is to prompt the lifestyle changes that will prevent cancer.

Sophie: Can you clarify how this is relevant to enhancement debate?

Eugenie: Certainly. The points that apply to the connection between genes and cancer also apply to the enhancement choices of a parent who chooses your DNA in accordance with their particular vision of the good life. Suppose your parents select genetic influences that they believe will make you a genius in mathematics. You learn of this and in a fit of pique dedicate yourself to writing poetry, refusing to ever look at a mathematical equation. No genetic modification is required for a child to thwart a parental plan to turn them into a genius in mathematics.

Sophie: I think I follow that. Perhaps there is no principled difference between the selection of genetic and environmental influences. But at what point does the child, or rather we on the child's behalf, get to say "Enough already!" There are so many societal pressures on today's children. Isn't the worry that by granting parents control over yet another influence on a child's development, we exceed a threshold of control? They already impart their views about the difference between right and wrong and choose the educational philosophy of their child's schooling. Now we're giving them control over their children's genomes. As the pressures mount what's left for the child?

Winston: I'm going to echo Sophie here. The educational pressures on today's children are already immense. Things are not as they were when we went to school. Our parents hoped that we come back from school doing basic arithmetic and knowing that in spelling it's "I before e, except after c." They trusted society to find good jobs for us and to provide the conditions for our flourishing. That's not how it is today. We're almost signing our kids up for vocational classes from the age of five. Now we are going to add genetic influences to this miasma of control? I think that what our age most needs right now is an updating of the lyrics of the Pink Floyd song. "Hey, genetic engineer, leave them kids alone!"

Eugenie: Enough of your maudlin nostalgia, Winston. Life back then wasn't perfect for everyone, you know. If I remember correctly you spent much of your schooling moaning about the pressures to academically excel.

Do we need enhancement tech risk pioneers?

Winston: Thanks Eugenie, perhaps I'm viewing my past through rose-tinted glasses. But let's take a break to mull this all over. I've long wanted to try absinthe, the alcoholic beverage once deemed so dangerous that it was banned in many parts of the world. There's a rumour that it causes hallucinations. Olen – can you promise me that the Metaverse plus neural lace version of absinthe will give me the fun stuff but protect me from any ill effects?

Olen: Sure! I've never tried absinthe and I certainly haven't tried to code it into the Metaverse. But why don't I assure you that it's perfectly safe and encourage you to give it a go. My hero Elon takes a fake-it-till-you-make-it approach to driverless car technology. So why not here too? Eugenie, do you mind if I take the lead in advocating the liberal view now?

Eugenie: Sure, but I'll be ready to interject if your suggestions conflict with a version of liberalism that I am happy with. Olen, you and I share a general endorsement of human enhancement, but I suspect that there is much that we disagree about regarding how societies regulate our enhancement choices.

Olen: I think we need what the philosopher Allen Buchanan refers to as "risk pioneers" – individuals prepared to experiment with exciting new technologies before the rest of us, who may be fearful, try them. We need some people to try virtual absinthe to confirm that it's safe for the rest of us. The same recommendation applies to enhancement technologies.

Winston: Thank for that carefully cautious endorsement of virtual absinthe, Olen. So you are inviting us to try it so that the company selling it to us can iron out any bugs? That raises a concern about the liberal arrangement that Eugenie and Olen seem to be advocating. We aren't just talking about philosophical arguments for enhancement. We should also be addressing commercial interests in enhancement technologies. Are you worried about the risks your enhancement risk pioneers are being encouraged to take? Companies are marketing barely tested technologies at us. Do you worry that many of the enhancements currently being sold on Amazon don't work? I suspect that many people who pay the high prices demanded on the Amazon Marketplace are being duped. Are they victims of an enhancement mania? This could be very profitable for corporate interests but predictably harmful for many purchasers of enhancement technologies.

Olen: I have more confidence that you in the wisdom of the crowd Winston. I can easily imagine a future time in a mature Age of Human Enhancement in which we view some of today's high-priced nootropics as fraudulent. But the beginning of the Age of Enhancement will be a time of exploration. Progress requires risk pioneers. Hardy folks risked everything to set sail from a miserable oppressive Europe. Some died. But survivors founded the New World.

Winston: Yes, that was good for some of those Europeans, but not so good for many people for whom the lands they discovered weren't "New."

Sophie: This seems to me to be a different concern you're raising here, Winston. You're clearly taking our discussion far beyond a focus on the specifics of gene editing.

Winston: I am a historian, aren't I? Historians are required to think broadly. I predict that I will be returning to the theme I've identified here of problems of enhancement technologies that are apparent only once we consider their broader social, historical, and economic contexts.

Olen: Fair enough Winston, but I think you get my point. Enhancement risk pioneers knowingly accept the risks of unproven enhancement tech. For that our descendants will owe them a debt of gratitude. They freely accept risks in an informed way and future generations get the gift of tested enhancement technologies. Those who safely travel by air today should be grateful to the risk pioneers who strapped themselves into the dangerous aeronautical contraptions of the early 1900s.

Winston: Yes, perhaps we will say thank you to the enhancement risk pioneers who willingly part with money to test nootropics and who volunteer themselves and their offspring to test the first attempts to use gene editing to enhance cognitive powers. Perhaps statues to He Jiankui will join statues of Christopher Columbus. Though, as with Columbus statues, what we think about these statues rather depends on how we think the Age of Human Enhancement has turned out. I would like to address that issue.

Eugenie, are you happy with Olen's extension of your view? Or do you think that he has hijacked it?

Eugenie: Unsurprisingly, I'm not nearly so enthusiastic about the wisdom of these risk pioneers that Olen is celebrating.

We've seen how eugenics can produce hideous outcomes if the state empowers experts in human heredity to choose what kinds of people get to exist. But I'm equally concerned about what will happen if we give undue control over our species' future to risk pioneers. Far too many people are lining up to invest their life savings in Elon Musk's companies. I worry about the consequences if Musk presents himself as a very charismatic risk pioneer for which ever enhancement technology one of his companies is selling.

Winston: (*his avatar grimaces ironically and points at the approximate location of the neural lace in its head*) I think I can see that risk. So what would your solution be to the undue influence of risk pioneers?

Eugenie: I want the liberal state to protect us against foolish choices. We have noted the evils that can be perpetrated by authoritarian states. But there is another risk that the Age of Human Enhancement brings. We've seen how charismatic tech people can lead many to make choices about investing in crypto currency that they come to regret. My version of the liberal state will seek to prevent foolish choices about enhancement technologies.

Is human enhancement a threat to equality?

Winston: I'm worried for the people who don't get access to these enhancements. Perhaps they can't afford them. Perhaps their parents chose not to use them. What do we say to the unenhanced human in the Age of Human Enhancement who missed out simply because their parents were either too poor or too religious, or both?

Eugenie: Liberal political philosophers have a response to that. They acknowledge your point and require that states should make enhancement technologies available as broadly as possible.

Winston: Thanks Eugenie, but there is a big gap between presenting an argument for the justice of distributing enhancement technologies broadly and acting as if the world *is* as we suppose it *should* be. There's a big gap between coming up with a sound argument for doing something about the climate crisis and actually doing something. Can you offer some reassurance, as we enter the Age of Human Enhancement with actual enhancement technologies, we won't soon arrive at the world described in Lee Silver's 1998 book *Remaking Eden: How Genetic Engineering and Cloning Will Transform the American Family*. Silver imagined the emerging genetic technologies of the 1990s transforming humanity into at least two distinct species – the enhanced GenRich and unenhanced Naturals. Perhaps some sensitive souls among the GenRich will understand that this polarization was regrettable. But they will be getting on with the world that they inherit. They will no more be able to stop this polarization then we can reverse the colonization of the "New" World that followed Columbus's "discovery" of it.

Eugenie: I wonder if you're making too much of this Winston. The goods of the Age of Human Enhancement aren't voided even if they aren't perfectly distributed according to your political ideals. How many people have access to this part of the Metaverse, for example? I looked at my credit card and was shocked by how much these virtual coffees are costing me.

Winston: I still have a concern about the consequences of unequal access to cognitive enhancement for inequality.

Eugenie: Please proceed. But please bear in mind that inequality is a moral challenge with a long history and political philosophers have thought hard about how best to address it.

Winston: Thank you, Eugenie. I have browsed those sections of the Great Library. Here's a new concern about inequality raised specifically by access to enhancement technologies that boost intelligence. We like to tell ourselves stories about the past in which we emphasize the importance of giving and understanding reasons.

Eugenie: Yes, I like that version of history too. People spent too long believing that they were allowed to own other human beings. But eventually they understood the reasons for the immorality of slavery. That's certainly an oversimplification of the history of slavery's demise. But I would like to think that it approximates to the truth.

Winston: Thanks Eugenie. I hope you are not ignoring the many human beings today who are effectively owned by others.

Eugenie: Sorry Winston. But there are certainly parts of the world where the immorality of slavery is now well understood. I don't expect political parties there to campaign on bringing back slavery.

Winston: Here's my concern about the creation of a society in which some people are beneficiaries of enhancement technologies, whilst others have missed out. It really would be a gross oversimplification of the past if we suppose that all slave owners abruptly "got" the immorality of owning other human beings and immediately freed their human chattels. Slave owners had invested large sums of money in the practice. They offered philosophical defences of it. For example, we now recognize claims that some humans are natural slaves as spurious. But this should not blind us to the fact that, at the time, these arguments defending slavery were offered in all earnestness, and by people who we think should have known better.

Eugenie: Sounds like you are making the case for moral progress. I'm all in favour of that. Surely cognitive enhancement will protect us and our descendants against reasoning that purports to justify slavery.

Winston: Perhaps we won't see the return of slavery. We should be grateful for that. But what about other varieties of injustice. Suppose we do see a separation of our descendants into cognitively enhanced GenRich and unenhanced Naturals. It may be that the GenRich are far too intellectually sophisticated to argue that they should be permitted to enslave the Naturals. But there are forms of ill-treatment beyond enslavement.

Sophie: What's your concern here? I'm sure that there are forms of injustice beyond slavery. But why do think that the Naturals are so likely to suffer them?

Winston: I'm concerned about the capacity of the Naturals to offer philosophically effective complaints about these future forms of injustice. They will be at a disadvantage when engaging in philosophical disputes with the enhanced GenRich. Imagine a past in which we gave defenders of slavery cognitive enhancement pills. They don't use their enhanced cognitive powers to recognize the wrongness of owning other human beings. Instead, they use their enhanced minds to mount very sophisticated defences of slavery.

Sophie: This all sounds a tad theoretical to me Winston. Can you give me an example?

Winston: I'm supposing you've followed the debates about gig work in today's digital economy. Some gig workers have offered effective complaints about their work conditions. What about a future in which the Natural gig workers find their philosophical objections all rebutted by GenRich employers who've chosen to focus on the benefits of the gig economy brought to the GenRich species or class? Part of the story about the end of slavery was the capacity of the enslaved to make powerful objections against their status. I am concerned that the Naturals' philosophical complaints may be viewed as no more philosophically persuasive than the bleats of sheep about to be slaughtered for our evening meals.

Sophie: This may seem like an odd response in a philosophical discussion. I've suggested that we use our imaginations to invent a wide range of thought experiments to test our theories. My concern about your thought experiment is that it refers to a possible future that is difficult for us to understand. Winston, you are asking us to imagine specific kinds of possible future GenRich people. These GenRich people want to treat Naturals in ways that seem unfair to us. Perhaps they don't want to enslave Naturals. But your gig work example suggests that you are worried that they may want to employ Naturals in other ways that seem unfair to us. They offer very sophisticated defences of this intuitively unfair treatment. They easily rebut the Naturals philosophical objections. Have I characterized your point correctly?

Winston: Yes.

Olen: Can I reply with a philosopher's version of "Show me the money!" – Show me the argument! Before I take your objection seriously I need more than a vague-sounding "Imagine an argument!"

Winston: I'm far from certain that this will happen. But Sophie encouraged us to not be overconfident about the future. Now that I've raised it as a possibility, can you give me some assurance that it won't happen, or if you can't, that you have thought through how this challenge might be met.

Sophie: Yes, it is a possibility that shouldn't just be dismissed.

Will human enhancement end sex?

Winston: There's so much to read about enhancement and the selection of hereditary material. Here's something a bit scandalous about what enhancement technologies could do to human reproduction. Suppose we take seriously the original idea of eugenics – that we should arrange the betterment of the race – or less controversially – the species.

Sophie: I thought that was your big complaint about Olen – too many tech fantasies about how future tech could effortlessly and unproblematically enhance us?

Winston: I've come across something by an Australian philosopher called Rob Sparrow that seems to be offering an outlandish thought experiment to make the opposite point. It's what philosophers refer to as a *reductio ad absurdum*. He explores the implications of a view that some bioethicists have advocated and aims to reduce them to absurdity. According to Sparrow, if you can't accept the consequence he describes you should reconsider your ethical endorsement of enhancement. His principal target is his fellow Australian Julian Savulescu who's one of the big current advocates of human enhancement. To use the lingo of Australian sporting clashes, this is very much a mate-versus-mate affair.

Eugenie: For the benefit of the rest of us, what's Savulescu's argument here?

Winston: He argues for a principle which seems allied to eugenic thinking – the Principle of Procreative Beneficence. According to this principle, given the choice of human lives to bring into existence, we are all subject to the moral obligation to choose the best one.

Sophie: I have located Savulescu's argument. The Principle directs that we choose the best embryo among those available. By best, he means the embryo that we expect to give rise to the life with the highest well-being.

Eugenie: So how does Savulescu imagine that we would arrange this choice?

Winston: His argument is most straightforwardly applied to reproductive technologies like IVF that can create many embryos. He thinks we would use a technology known as Pre-Implantation Diagnosis to analyse the DNA of each of these embryos. We then look for genetic variants that predictably reduce or increase expected well-being and use that information to guide our choices about which to implant in a future mother's womb. This is an existing technology and it is already used to enable parents at risk of passing on a serious genetic disease to avoid doing so.

Eugenie: Perhaps you can give us an example.

Winston: Consider the serious developmental disorder Lesch-Nyhan syndrome. It's inherited and mostly affects males, resulting in a variety of negative effects on well-being. These include, most notably, obsessive self-mutilating behaviours such as lip and finger biting and head banging. It's a recessive disorder meaning that for it to be passed on, a child must inherit two copies of the Lesch-Nyhan genetic variant. Pre-Implantation Diagnosis enables women to avoid pregnancies with embryos that have two copies of the genetic variant.

Eugenie: I think I can see how the Principle extends beyond avoiding genetic disease. Genomic studies are revealing genetic variants linked with variation in well-being. There are genetic variants that make people more or less euthymic, where "euthymia" is the state of having a tranquil mental state or mood. So the Principle of Procreative Beneficence would require that your pregnancy begin with the embryo that has genetic variants linked with euthymia rather than dysthymia which has the opposite effect on well-being. People who are dysthymic may not satisfy clinical definitions of depression, but they are predictably less happy than euthymic people. So why are you, of all people, presenting this case to us, Winston? Are you joining team enhancement?

Winston: That does sound quite a lot like the eugenics as originally described by Galton. Talk about moral requirements seems to make it different from liberal eugenics. But Rob Sparrow has a response to the view.

Olen: More philosophical negativity about exciting new tech? I think I'm not going to like this. What's Sparrow's response?

Winston: Suppose there really is an obligation to create the human life with the highest well-being. If so, given the kind of choice imagined by Savulescu, shouldn't we prefer female embryos to male embryos?

Olen: Why's that? I'm male and I'm doing very well, thank you. Did I tell you that my social media start-up is now a unicorn with a market valuation of over one billion dollars? That's US dollars, not the crummy New Zealand coin that Agar gets paid in.

Winston: Yes, I think you told us that, Olen. But reminders are always useful. Sparrow gives reasons for thinking that a female embryo should be expected to give rise to an embryo with higher well-being than a male embryo. Now that females have been liberated from an obligation to have as many children as possible, they live longer than males.

Sophie: I see that – certainly in economically advanced nations women do, on average, outlive men.

Winston: Sparrow cites another benefit of being female. Women get to bring new lives into existence. They aren't restricted to the adjunct sperm-providing roles of males.

Sophie: Now that is a twist. I'm not sure what to make of that claim. Can I just clarify the gender of Sparrow? He is male isn't he? As a woman I've long been committed to the cause of women's control over our reproductive capacities. The right to have an abortion is a central element of that. One of the supposed benefits of the sexual revolution in the 1960s and 1970s was that everyone got to enjoy causal sex. I'm all in favour of that but women tended to get stuck with the consequences. Do I hear Sparrow correctly when he seemingly suggests that we shouldn't complain so much about that?

Winston: How so, Sophie?

Sophie: Well, if pregnancy is this wonderful gift then is he saying we shouldn't complain so much about the downside of occasional unwanted pregnancies. I'm thinking of an analogy …

Winston: Let's hear it.

Sophie: Well, there are some irritations to being rich. If you own a mansion you may have to pay annoying property

Winston: taxes. But we don't feel too sorry for the rich if they get to live in the mansions, they are more than compensated for the irritating taxes.

Winston: You'll have to explain this to me, Sophie. So pregnancies are mansions in this story?

Sophie: It is an analogy. I'm just imagining Sparrow's Grandad approaching marchers for the right to terminate a pregnancy with the response "What are you moaning about? You are so much more fortunate than me – I can't get pregnant. Why can't you put up with carrying the occasional unwanted pregnancy to full-term? After all many pregnancies are joyfully wanted."

Winston: I'm sure Sparrow wouldn't say that!

Olen: Time for a round of virtual absinthes!

Is liberal eugenics just shit stirring?

Winston: I'm experiencing an increasing sense of unease about this whole discussion. We've been discussing how "liberal" this version of eugenics is. But now I'm wondering about the motivation for this whole view. What motivated philosophers to formulate this liberal eugenics and advocate it? I think I understood what a liberal view about genetic selection would be. Is this just that view with the word "eugenics" thrown in to get attention?

Eugenie: So you are accusing Agar and me of philosophically impure motives?

Winston: Indeed! Liberal eugenics attracts attention because it's an oxymoron. Everyone should know about the offences committed in the name of eugenics. Now they find someone advocating it by simply appending the word liberal. After this, what comes next? Why not philosophical defences of Nice Nazis? We would clarify that the "nice" part suggests no endorsement of Nazi views about genocide. No, Nice Nazis reject genocide, murder of the disabled, wars of aggression, and everything associated with those evils. Nice Nazis are into the sharp fashions of Hugo Boss-designed uniforms and the precision engineering that made excellent jet fighters. Nice Nazis take credit for the world's first public health campaign against smoking.

Sophie: Perhaps I can help out here. I think you're accusing Eugenie of doing something worse than advancing a provocative oxymoron. You are accusing her of philosophical shit stirring.

Olen: What!? Sophie, I thought you'd made a point about the importance of civility in our philosophical discussions. Now profanity is allowed?

Sophie: Philosophical shit stirring is a technical term. It is inspired by another philosophically principled scatological reference. The American thinker Harry Frankfurt introduced the concept of bullshitting to philosophers. His 1986 article "On Bullshit" opens with the great line that "One of the most salient features of our culture is that there is so much bullshit." This short article caused a bit of discussion at the time. But it enjoyed a philosophical resurgence with the presidency of Donald Trump. Trump turned out to have a special talent for bullshitting.

Olen: Sophie, please tell me you're not going to subject us to another of your prolonged academic philosopher's expressions of disdain for Trump. He's no longer president!

Sophie: I'll spare you that. But Trump does turn out to be the perfect embodiment of bullshitting. According to Frankfurt bullshitting is different from lying which involves deliberately passing falsehood off as truth.

Olen: So how's that relevant to Trump?

Sophie: When responding to the pandemic Trump often made statements that turned out to be false. Remember his assertion that coronavirus could be cured by introducing a very powerful bright light into the body. This was false but I don't think he knew enough about the virus to know that it was false. So he wasn't really lying. I suspect he hoped that it was true. He found himself giving a press conference in which journalists had many questions about the COVID-19 and he chose to bullshit. There were plenty of people whom he could have asked – Deborah Birx, the White House Coronavirus Response Coordinator, was in the room. If Trump had been interested in the truth he would have asked but instead he chose to pay no attention an authority of the truth about COVID-19. He bullshitted.

Olen: OK enough of your snooty disdain for the former president. What's shit stirring?

Sophie: Shit stirring stands to earnest advice as bullshitting stands to the truth. We can start with an Oxford English Dictionary definition. (*Sophie gestures and the OED definition of shit stirring appears.*)

To shit stir is "To attempt to provoke or aggravate, esp. without serious intent."

In ethics, shit stirring involves speech acts that have the grammatical form of advice but where there is no intent to provide useful advice, advice that recipients can or should act on.

Olen: Can you give us an example from outside of the moral domain?

Sophie: OK (*patting Olen on his balding head*). Olen, have you ever thought about getting hair plugs?

Olen: What!? I ask a perfectly innocent question and you insult me. I know that I'm losing my hair. I don't need you to verbally poke me like that. And no, I don't want hair plugs. But I think maybe that you know that.

Sophie: You see what I did there? My speech act had the grammatical form of advice. But of course, it was just a verbal poke. And your response proves my point. I got a rise out of you. It seems to me that calling a liberal view about human enhancement "eugenics" is just a poke. It's designed to aggravate people. Agar, the dude who combined the eugenics with liberal even confessed that the view is a philosophical shit stir. This particular shit stir had its desired effect. We've been talking about Habermas. Well, that eminent German philosopher was so annoyed that he expressed his annoyance at a 1998 presentation of liberal eugenics in his 2003 book. Apparently, Agar's view summed up much that was wrong about the Anglo-Saxon liberal approach to the new genetic technologies. Having Habermas criticize him was certainly excellent for Agar's academic citation count. So that's a philosophical shit-stirrer's mission accomplished.

Winston: There can be negative effects from shit stirring about human reproduction. There is renewed attention to the historic crimes of eugenics. We may think that eugenics is a thing of the past. But eugenic attitudes persist and continue to harm those assessed as hereditarily inferior.

Eugenie: I think I need a virtual absinthe after that! Let's take a break to look out the window and view this presentation of 1890s London.

The friends wander over to the window. After half an hour of scrutiny of virtual inhabitants of late nineteenth century London they return.

Eugenie: (*in an indignant voice*) Sorry but I think Agar's confession is mistaken. Liberal eugenics is not a shit stir. It's useful. It's useful even if it is mistaken in some of its philosophical details. Here's why you should be grateful for this linguistic novelty even if you think the view is philosophically mistaken.

Winston: So I should be happy about Agar's focus on his citation count? I very much doubt that. These are serious issues here. We are talking about how powerful technologies may affect – or corrupt – human nature.

Sophie: I think I can see Eugenie's point. We may think we have progressed far beyond Galton's racist misunderstandings. We should acknowledge that eugenics was, nevertheless, the first scientifically informed attempt to enhance humans. Perhaps this is the true philosophical value of Agar's and Eugenie's advocacy of liberal eugenics. Terrible offences were perpetrated in the name of eugenics. When the Nazis murdered almost 300,000 disabled people, that was eugenics. We need constant reminders of that crime so as to avoid making the same errors. A modern label such as "a liberal view about genetic modification" promotes a dangerous forgetting in which we assume that because we have updated our scientific understandings of heredity we are guaranteed to avoid such errors in the future. We are less likely to be alerted to historical moral offences if some advocate says "our liberal approach to genetic technologies requires that they not be offered to people with a significant disability because of the high cost to the state of offering them" than if the advocate says "according to liberal eugenics we shouldn't offer genetic services to the disabled."

Winston: Eugenie, are you happy with Sophie's philosophical finessing of your view? Or are you going to accuse *her* of philosophically shit stirring you! She's in effect saying that liberal eugenics is great, not because it's the correct view, but because keeping the term around helps people to not repeat historical mistakes. Are you happy with that "possibly bad but certainly useful" evaluation of your view, Eugenie?

Eugenie: Actually, I think I'm fine with it. I'm not an overconfident philosopher. We are making claims about the future – how future technologies, many of which are yet to be invented, could be used. Saying that eugenics is simply morally right or morally wrong leaves us ill-prepared for an uncertain future. I choose to view eugenics as essentially morally problematic. We are making choices about which kinds of human beings – or, if I can venture a prediction about where Olen wants to take this conversation, posthumans – get to exist. Moral problems like this can't be straightforwardly solved in the way take some scientific problems are. People in earlier times wondered about the geological composition of the Moon. Now we know. It's been removed from our list of problems. We will *never* remove questions about how to make the next generation of humans – or posthumans – from that list. I'm betting that there won't be a time in the future at which we can look at enhancement choices as simply morally wrong or simply morally right. By preserving the term eugenics we ensure that when future generations try to solve these problems they look as far back as the earliest attempts to use science to decide what kinds of people should exist. Liberal eugenics offers insurance against dangerous forgetting. We know that authoritarian eugenics as recommended by Galton and practiced by Hitler's racial experts is wrong. But we must be constantly alert to the reintroduction of its moral mistakes into our liberal view.

Olen: I'm not sure about you guys, but I found this historical tour a bit depressing. I really needed the virtual alcohol! The exciting future of an enhanced humanity can't be all about being terrified of reinstating Hitler and Himmler and their coterie of evil race scientists. Tomorrow evening we are going to look at the exciting future offered by enhancement technologies.

Sophie: I suspect you are best placed to decide where we conduct that discussion, Olen.

Night 4   Radical versus moderate enhancement and cognition

Coffee on the bridge of USS Enterprise *(NCC-1701-D)*

Winston: OK Olen, so where are we now?

Olen: We are on the bridge of USS *Enterprise* (NCC-1701-D), the *Enterprise* of *Star Trek: The Next Generation*. I picked this place to have virtual coffee to counteract some of the doom and gloom of last night's discussion. Somehow you guys took something beautiful – all about improving humanity – and turned it into something abhorrently racist and evil. I thought coffee on the bridge of Jean Luc Picard's *Enterprise* was the place to revive the optimistic can-do attitude that characterizes humanity's best instincts. Let's move away from thoughts about retro concepts like eugenics and consider what human beings could become if we were imaginative about how to apply to our human natures some of the techs that *Star Trek* creator Gene Roddenberry placed on his twenty-fourth century starship.

Winston: No surprises there. You've always been a Trekkie. Now you're going to use enhancement technologies to make Roddenberry's 1960s fantasy real!

Olen: Not so fast, Winston. I want to highlight one respect in which Roddenberry wasn't far-sighted enough. Sophie, you've already shit-stirred me about my hair loss. In the 2500s the humans who travel the galaxy won't look anything like the bald Patrick Stewart, unless of course

DOI: 10.4324/9781003321613-4

they choose to. And yes, I would like to add a cure for male pattern balding to the list of patches for humanity that will take us far beyond what we today accept as normal.

Sophie: So Olen, after a fix for baldness, what comes next?

A radically enhanced humanity remade by tech?

Winston: I can see that we've come some way beyond Galton's proposal to manage human reproduction. But let me repeat Santayana's line "Those who cannot remember the past are condemned to repeat it." I want to suggest a barrier that arises in respect of the digital techs that Olen is about to propose that we apply to our human natures. We are dazzled by technological novelties and this hampers our ability to learn from history. Many of Galton's proposals seem patently wrong to us today. But we mustn't overlook the fact that those who first encountered them viewed them as fresh teachings about humanity's future from the thrilling new science of evolution.

Eugenie: This sounds like the beginning of a Winston rant!

Winston: Thanks Eugenie, but I'm just trying to make the point that every age's inventions seem to them to be entirely and excitingly new. They seem to offer advantages unknown to the science and technology of earlier ages. They also seem to dodge all the moral challenges that beset past technologies. Shiny iPhones are cool and we forget that they are essentially similar to the communications technologies that preceded them. We too easily forget the lessons learned about past techs.

Olen: (*groans*) So, you're determined to drag us back to nasty authoritarian eugenics?

Winston: That's the only good thing about this horrid liberal eugenics, IMHO. People like you, Olen, want us to forget the past. It's true that no one trying to sell brain-boosting nootropics on the Amazon Marketplace would think to market their products as the latest development of positive eugenics. But perhaps it would be helpful if they did. Maybe they should be required to as a prompt to remember history's moral teachings. Mind you, it's hard to imagine Amazon.com Inc. enforcing that! I'm thinking that the same racist impulses that Galton made explicit will find ways to guide our application of nootropics, gene editing, and cybernetics.

Sophie: Olen, I can accept that these enhancement techs could be very powerful. Perhaps you can shed some light on that. I seem to remember that most of the crew of the NCC-1701-D looked pretty much like us.

Olen: And here we come to the annoying aspect of my favourite show. We are supposed to accept that they travelled at many times the speed of light, but they looked pretty much like ordinary human beings of the 1990s. We have the android Data. But, except for a storyline about an evil twin Lore, Data is an outlier. He's so obviously smarter and stronger than his human crewmates – and much better adapted to space. Data doesn't need to suit up for spacewalks. If we cast our imaginations forward, the spacefaring humans of the twenty-fourth century will almost certainly have integrated much of Data's tech into their brains and bodies. They won't be a different caste of robotic beings. They will be us.

Winston: Can we please not treat this discussion as another opportunity for you to express your Trekkie identity?

Olen: Duly noted. But if we really are launching photon torpedoes in the twenty-fourth century, we won't look anything like the very unenhanced human William Shatner who played Captain James Tiberius Kirk in the 1960s series. We won't look like the bald Patrick Stewart who played Jean-Luc Picard in the 1990s series – my favourite *Star Trek* series by the way. We will have benefited from a wide range of genetic, cybernetic, and nootropic enhancements. Yes, Sophie, we will have fixed baldness.

Winston: I really don't want to interrupt your sales pitch. But what will we look like?

Olen: I bet that we will look more like creatures re-engineered to survive and thrive in space. The finishing touches of the evolution of our current bodies and psyches were orchestrated in the Holocene, an epoch in Earth's history that commenced 11,700 years ago. Adaptations that worked for that epoch won't protect us against the disruptions of the stable Holocene from our misuse of the technologies of the Industrial Revolution. We are now having to deal with the environmental consequences of the economic growth generated by the steam engine.

Sophie: Your selection of the bridge of USS *Enterprise* suggests that there's more to your pro-enhancement spiel than protecting us against climate change.

Olen: Correct. But there turns out to be a link between going into space and protecting against climate change.

Sophie: So what's wrong with space-faring humans in the twenty-fourth century looking much like us? When I see paintings of humans in the seventeenth century they look pretty familiar to me.

Olen: The notion of twenty-fourth century humans travelling into space with the unenhanced biology of the Pleistocene is about as absurd as supposing that you can take on a Borg Cube with a catapult that hurls the stones that the ancient Romans used to scare away the barbarians of 100 CE. I am thinking that the changes to humanity that equip us for space will reach deeper than our skins. Occasionally in *Star Trek: The Next Generation* we got to see Data's positronic brain. I suspect that space-faring humans won't entirely delete our biological brains. But a scan of the brains of the space-faring humans of the twenty-fourth century would reveal many digital enhancements seamlessly integrated with vestigial biological brain matter. Granted, they're unlikely to look much like the flashing lights of Data's positronic brain.

Winston: Perhaps I don't want to become a space-faring posthuman. I have to confess that the scenes in *Star Trek* that most inspired me were those in which Captain Picard retreats to harvest grapes in Burgundy. If we respond to the challenge of climate change, can't we hope to make that kind of pleasant, distinctively human life available to more of us?

Olen: Winston, I'm with you on the importance of responding to climate change and other extinction threats. But these should involve going into space too. I'm sorry to say that there is a limit to the number of humans who can lead the idyllic wine-making existence that *Star Trek* occasionally presents Picard as enjoying. I think we should follow Elon Musk's plan as he presented it in 2021 – "We don't want to be one of those single-planet species; we want to be a multi-planet species." Our biologies worked well for the Earthly conditions for which we evolved. Our irresponsible contributions to climate change messed that up somewhat. The unfriendly human environment that we are creating will soon necessitate some technological upgrades for humanity. But if we want to go into space, or to live in the deranged environment of the Anthropocene and not just barely survive, but thrive, we will need to forsake much of our cumbersome Pleistocene-designed biology.

Sophie: OK Olen. Suppose we accept that powerful technologies will be applied to our obsolete brains and bodies. Are we just supposed to accept that any way tech remakes us will be good?

Olen: Look, I'm not as obsessively limited by history as Winston seems to be. I'm an optimist who always thinks that we can do better. But I certainly know enough to understand that powerful technologies can be misused. However, don't worry. There's a fix. If we are going to use these powerful technologies well, we need to morally enhance ourselves. But more on that later.

Winston: Whenever tech people talk about fixes for big problems I always suspect a scam. We hear so much reckless talk about tech fixes. But the subtext always seems to be "Relax, don't worry! Do nothing!" You could make the painful sacrifices required to curb carbon emissions. Or you could do nothing and await the supercool climate techs of 2035. These will clean up all past, present, and future carbon emissions and permit us to proceed on our current gas-guzzling ways. That's the message I took out of Bill Gates's 2021 book, *How to Avoid a Climate Disaster*. Gates did talk about the need to make sacrifices, but he also pushed these amazing future climate techs that would seemingly render painful curbs on emissions pointless.

Differences between liberal eugenics and radical enhancement

Olen: There you go again, Winston, changing the topic again. Enough virtue-signalling about climate change. We are talking about human enhancement. There are three areas of improvement that most excite me as we enter the Age of Human Enhancement. One area of enhancement is cognitive. We need to apply tech to our brains. The COVID-19 pandemic pushed our species to its limit. We are going to need to be a lot smarter to respond to future challenges that may be even nastier than COVID-19.

Winston: Thinking back on my memory of growing up with you, I'm not surprised that you're interested in getting smarter. Has your science officer Spock impression gotten any better?

Olen: *(beginning to look annoyed and adopting a sarcastic tone)* Thanks Winston! But enhancement technologies offer so much more than additional IQ points. There's also the promise of life extension. We seem to have hit a hard upper limit to how far healthy diets and lifestyles can take us. We need to apply tech to our crummy human biology. Today we look at all the exciting things offered by an increasingly technological future, but we believe that we will never get to actually see and experience them. Starships shouldn't be only for our descendants. Let's live long enough to be on them.

Winston: (*Winston's avatar sneers*) Hmm, I really can't think how any of this could go wrong ...

Olen: But wait, there's more. Not only will we be *much* smarter and live *much* longer we will also be happier, *much* happier. Winston, I remember that prolonged depressed phase you went through at university. How did you move past that?

Winston: Yes, that was difficult. I wonder if it might have been partly connected with coming out as gay. Thanks for remembering, Olen. Coming out did help in the end, but I did make heavy use of the university counselling services and of antidepressants.

Olen: You seem so much better now. But it turns out that many normally happy people struggle with moods that are lower than they could be. There are differences between the hyperthymic – those among us who are naturally more joyful, interested, and content – and the rest of us. Winston, you are clearly no longer clinically depressed, but could you not be happier? The great thing is that there are drugs that can help and the promise of more powerful drugs in the near future.

Winston: Thank you for your concern, Olen. But I don't think I need your drugs.

Olen: Well ... even if you're no longer clinically depressed, you have become a bit of a curmudgeon. Perhaps a well-targeted pharmaceutical might help you to be a bit more optimistic about the world that enhancement technologies could make.

Sophie: How's this different from Eugenie's liberal view? Eugenie's approach to our enhanced future was inspired by Galton's plan to manage human reproduction. If I remember correctly she transferred enhancement choices from the state to individual procreators. How is what you're saying different?

Eugenie: Yes Olen, just to add my voice to Sophie's sceptical query, when we look at the enhancement produced by the evolutionary process we can see that Galton's plan to shape humanity could work, its many moral offences notwithstanding. All I hear from you, Olen, is a pitch grounded in exaggerated hopes for future tech. When I watch *Star Trek* I watch it as science *fiction*. For you, it seems to be a window into the future. Your main interest seems to be to fix those occasional respects in which it wasn't crazy enough about what humanity could become.

Olen: Thanks Eugenie … Not! I hereby declare our pro-enhancement philosophical alliance over. Your retro enhancement plan would graft a few new techs on to Galton's evolutionary mechanism. I'm committed to realizing the full potential of new technologies, especially new digital ones.

Winston: I'm worried that you are too easily duped by the chutzpah of tech visionaries. If I hear you right, there won't be any baldness in the future and we will be able to go on spacewalks without the need for cumbersome spacesuits. You've been gulled by the marketing of tech types like Elon Musk. Musk's billions are testament to his talent at selling us, and investors, exciting visions of future tech. There's nothing that violates the laws of logic or physics in stories about driverless cars that outperform human drivers. But Musk's 2020 deadline is well passed and I don't see those cars. To what extent is our excitement about future enhancement technologies really little more than a tribute to our regrettable urge to unthinkingly reach for tech solutions to our toughest problems?

Olen: Here's my concern about Eugenie's go slow approach. Galton's programme of managed reproduction suggests that enhanced intellects and extended lifespans might take a long time to arrive. I don't think you will speed up the arrival of an enhanced future all that much if you use gene editing to tweak a gene or two, here and there. We need to enlist fast-improving digital technologies and direct them at our obsolete human natures.

Winston: Can I ask what's the hurry? I'm clearly more impressed by our human natures than you are, Olen. But I accept that they are changing and that the ever-changing technologies that fill our environments are much of the reason. I accept that change today occurs more rapidly than anything our ancestors experienced. But for you this change isn't fast enough. You seem to want to snap your fingers and significantly enhance us ASAP.

Olen: Yes, but this is more than the expression of tech mania that you seem to be suggesting. We need to get smarter faster. To follow up on your concern about the environment, there are too many empowered human beings who fail to grasp the scientific case for disastrous anthropocentric climate change. One of the reasons we didn't promptly deal with the SARS-Cov-2 virus was that too many of us failed to understand that very rare fatal side effects from vaccination don't make vaccines unsafe. Great-great-grandchildren intelligent enough to understand that speedy vaccination will protect us against COVID-79 won't be much use if COVID-29 has already sent us extinct. It's not just the case that we need to get smarter sooner. We need to get *much* smarter, *far* sooner. We need to unlock as much of the enhancement potential of genetic, cybernetic, and pharmacological technologies as we can.

Winston: I wonder how new this view that Olen is presenting really is. The philosopher Susan Levin argues that this transhumanist vision isn't as new as transhumanists suggest. She traces the view back to World War II. It's not all about new technologies. Rather it has a long history of failing to measure up to expectations.

Olen: Even if Levin is correct about the disappointments of the past we could surely be right this time. Let's not put too much faith in inductive reasoning which any philosopher should know is unsound. This time we're really going to deliver on our promises.

Radical human enhancement clarified

Sophie: Can you define what it is that you think humanity most needs? You can't expect us to accept the vague sounding notion that rather than just human enhancement, we need a *lots of* human enhancement. Can you take us beyond the definitions of enhancement that we heard about in the Great Library?

Olen: Sure Sophie. What we need is *radical* human enhancement. Radical enhancement is best illustrated by means of examples. I'm going to focus on two varieties – radical cognitive enhancement and radical life extension. But I am not oblivious to the concerns of my favourite sceptic Sophie, who insists on playing the philosopher's role of trying to catch me out with tough and annoying questions at every opportunity, and Winston who seems to be to be a bioconservative dedicated to keeping humans as stupid and short-lived as he can.

Sophie: OK Olen, we've heard your sales pitch. Now for the philosophical detail. What is *radical* enhancement supposed to be?

Olen: Thanks Sophie. Remember the two definitions of enhancement we discussed in the Great Library? There was one that identified enhancement with improvement. That definition seemed to make human enhancement good by definition. Who disagrees with people who seek to improve themselves? But there is another definition that seems more to the liking of bioconservatives like Winston. This account indexes enhancement to the biologically normal range of human abilities.

I'm going to pinch this definition, its obnoxious moral associations notwithstanding, to define radical enhancement. *Moderate* human enhancement improves its subjects within or just beyond the normal biological range for humans. *Radical* enhancement improves capacities to levels far beyond that range. A nootropic that that boosts an IQ from 110 to 120 would be a moderate enhancement. It's not a therapy simply because an IQ of 110 is beyond the average for human beings, which is, by definition 100. You might complain to your doctor that you would like to be more intelligent, but you wouldn't expect your doctor to prescribe therapies to treat the mental illness of having an IQ of 110 in the same way that they might prescribe an antidepressant to treat clinical depression. Your doctor might direct you to a nootropic sold on the Amazon Marketplace but that would be an enhancement and not a therapy. A neuroimplant that granted powers of focus far beyond the capacities of the best unenhanced human mind would be radical enhancement.

Winston: This assumes that we accept IQ tests as a measure of human cognitive abilities.

Olen: I understand that this is controversial. But for the time being can we accept this as an example that should serve the purposes of our philosophical debate. Even if you reject IQ as a measure of intelligence, you should at least accept that there is variation in human cognitive capacity. Some people are more intelligent than others. And there is no reason to believe that there is an upper limit. Even Albert Einstein could have been more intelligent.

Eugenie: I follow that, but this nevertheless sounds disappointingly vague. How do you determine where the category of radical enhancement begins? Boosting an IQ from

140 to 180 may sound like radical enhancement to some but not to others.

Olen: It's true that the boundaries between moderate and radical enhancement are vague. That may offend the tidy minds of analytic philosophers. But it's no problem if that vagueness exists in nature. Sophie, you mocked me for my premature balding – thanks for that ... And yes, I am placing male pattern baldness on my list of aspects of normal human existence that need fixing, albeit somewhat low. Since you've made my hair a topic of discussion I'm going to use it to illustrate a philosophical point. Sophie, would you say that I'm bald?

Sophie: Sorry about all the teasing – it was a long day in Francis Galton's musty study. But I can accept that though you are clearly suffering hair loss, you aren't bald.

Olen: Would you also agree that there is no precise dividing line between the bald and not bald? The boundary between these two states is imprecise and vague. Someone with zero hair follicles is straightforwardly bald. Someone with lots of hair is certainly not bald. But in between these clear categories are individuals like me, on the way to baldness, but not there yet.

Sophie: You're saying it's the same with the boundary between moderate and radical enhancement?

Olen: Yes Sophie. There is no result on an IQ test that marks the precise boundary between a moderately enhanced intellect and a radically enhanced one. There is no precise age or life expectancy that marks the boundary between a moderately extended life span and a radically extended one. Those boundaries are vague. But that shouldn't prevent us from talking about radically enhanced intellects just as we can talk about bald people.

Eugenie: Suppose that I accept your deliberately vague definitions, Olen. You joined this discussion as an enthusiast about the possibilities of applying digital technologies

	to our natures. Some of the examples you have given involve grafting digital technologies to our bodies. Is this part of your definition? Are radical enhancements just enhancements achieved by digital technologies?
Olen:	No Eugenie. Radical enhancements are defined as improvements of our capacities to levels far beyond the biologically normal range for human beings. But there is an interesting connection with digital technologies. As we will see, the most effective way to achieve great degrees of human enhancement is likely to be by applying digital technologies to our natures. Remember the examples that we used to introduce enhancement technologies. There were pharmacological, genetic, and cybernetic enhancements. Pharmacological and genetic improvements are likely to fall within the category of moderate enhancement. Cybernetic improvement involves the direct application of digital technologies to our natures. As we will see there are good reasons to think that this method of improving human beings will tend to bring many radical enhancements.
Winston:	This still sounds like science fantasy to me. Are we really going to waste our time debating whether it would be so much better to have an IQ of a trillion than a billion? I follow the point about one number being bigger than the other. But how will this help us to make wise choices about how we apply to our natures technologies that may be imminently available?
Olen:	Here's where things get very interesting. Prepare yourselves for some exciting tech offers!

Should we become posthuman?

Sophie:	I think I understand your enthusiasm about this radically enhanced future. I'm now experiencing quite nasty toothache and will have to duck out of the conversation for an emergency visit to my dentist. I understand that

dentistry isn't top of your tech wish list, Olen, but do you think we might get a future free of dental pain?

Olen: Yes, that's certainly on offer. Human teeth are another example of biological hardware good enough for the Pleistocene but nowhere near good enough for our enhanced descendants or, supposing we do fast-forward human enhancement, our enhanced future selves. I have to confess that I haven't thought much about it, but how about a future in which we integrate self-repair capacities into our teeth? Perhaps dental stem cells could be genetically edited to swiftly replace any damaged or diseased dental matter. Of course, if you're not attached to the pulp, dentine, enamel, and cementum that human teeth are currently made from then so many other possibilities open up ...

Winston: What, cyborg teeth? It's all so easy isn't it, Olen. You visit Wikipedia or turn on the Sci-Fi channel, see some cool future tech stuff and then start riffing. All I'm saying to Sophie is that you don't delay your emergency trip to the dentist just because Olen enjoys speculating about how applying future digital technologies to dental stem cells should promptly produce shiny, pain-free cyborg chompers.

Sophie: I have a booking. But before I go, will you permit me one further question? I like the idea of a future without dental pain. But I acknowledge the challenge to our humanity that may come from this. Perhaps the concern about losing our humanity would be addressed if you could give us a sense of where we are collectively headed. I'm sure it won't end with cyborg teeth, which right now I'd definitely sign up for. Will we still be human once we've accepted all of the enhancement tech offers that you have for us, Olen?

Winston: Yes, thank you Sophie. I strongly suspect that Olen is setting us up to be scammed. First we accept that we need cyborg teeth. What's next? We invest in some cryptocurrency and that makes us all fabulously wealthy? But suppose these enhancement technologies do promptly arrive, what happens to our humanity? I think I've made clear that the thing that you have contempt for, I cherish. Will we have laid waste to our human natures in exchange for some tech promises that are never honoured?

Olen: (*Olen's avatar pouts frustratedly*) Enough of your rhetoric Winston! There are no TV cameras here. It's just us. I am not convinced that we will lose our humanity. I see enhancement as the purest expression of the enlightenment ideal of humanity. Steven Pinker's 2018 book *Enlightenment Now* challenges the pessimism about progress that seems to have become entrenched in certain academic circles. Pinker looks back to the Enlightenment, a period of European history in the seventeenth and eighteenth centuries in which people increasingly sought to go beyond the revealed wisdom of their holy books and to seek solutions from reason and science. Pinker thinks that there has been a loss of faith in the enlightenment ideal. But scientific progress continues to massively improve human lives. The members of the thinkeratti enjoy questioning the value of mRNA vaccines, but think how many lives they saved as we've faced the challenges of COVID-19.

Winston: I hear and understand this celebration of scientific progress. But please let's not forget that Pinker is also the Harvard brain who told us, in that 2018 book, that these days "disease outbreaks don't become pandemics." Anyway, what does Pinker's celebration of societal and technological progress have to do with human enhancement?

Olen: Well, Pinker doesn't really go there. But the Swedish transhumanist philosopher Nick Bostrom certainly does. He presents great degrees of human enhancement as expressions of that enlightenment ideal. We solve the problems of nature by applying technology to them. We also apply these technologies to our Pleistocene-designed human natures and get even better at solving nature's problems. To put things in the terms we've just introduced, radical enhancement is the most emphatic continuation of the enlightenment ideal. The radical improvement of our technologies and ourselves is at the core of what it means to be human.

Winston: Can you stop speechifying, Olen!

Olen: Sorry, but I wanted to leave you in no doubt about the value of giving enhancement technologies free range to improve us. You and your fellow bioconservatives believe in a future in which things may change around us but we remain static. But that is the denial of our humanity which has always been about using our intellects to improve our circumstances and our lives.

Sophie: (*rubbing her jaw in pain*) Olen, can you tell us what, if we are no longer human, we will be? I accept that space travel complete with spacewalks that we can do without the need for anything like the Apollo spacesuit that Neil Armstrong wore for his moonwalk would be great. But I do want some sense of where we are all supposed to be going collectively.

Olen: Sure! We will become posthuman. According to the transhumanist FAQ

"a posthuman is a hypothetical future being whose basic capacities so radically exceed those of present humans as to be no longer unambiguously human by our current standards."

I propose that the relationship between humans and posthumans should be viewed as similar to the relationship between prehumans and humans. Here's one way to think about this. Humans are not prehumans. But we are *of* prehumans, in the sense that we came from them. There is an important relationship between us and them even if that relationship is not identity. We care about where we as a species came from in precisely the way the popularity of ancestry tracking sites demonstrate that there is money to be made telling people where they come from as individuals. The big market for books by evolutionary anthropologists, offering us theories about which species of hominins hanging out in Africa three million years ago *Homo sapiens* evolved from, supports that strong collective evaluative interest. We buy books that promise to tell humans where we collectively came from. The specific species or genus from which we evolved matters to us in a way that other species that happened to be hanging out in Africa at the same time as those direct ancestors don't. We have a similar collective interest in the beings who will predictably replace us. These posthumans will be *of* humans even if they definitely aren't human. We will care about them.

Sophie: This abstract philosophical theorising is both hurting my head and aggravating my toothache. So your revised position is that the beings that result from unrestricted application of enhancement technologies to ourselves *may* not be human but perhaps that won't matter so much if they are *of* us, where the "of" expresses an important evaluative relationship?

Olen: Nick Bostrom offers crisp exposition of that evaluative relationship with his line "Why I Want to be a Posthuman When I Grow Up." It will be us as humans who are growing up and turning into something so much better.

Sophie: My toothache is getting worse, but I think I'm ready to hear more of the scientific story about how we might become posthuman.

Olen: Sure Sophie. Let me reassure you that help is fast arriving for your tooth! Pain-free cyber-teeth will arrive more quickly than you think if we let digital technologies do their thing.

What is exponential technological progress?

Winston: Uh-oh. Something tells me we are about to take a techie tour of exponential technological progress and Moore's Law. Go on Olen, which story about exponential improvement are you going to tell us? The one about the inventor who asks the king to pay him by placing one grain of rice on the first square of a chess board, two grains on the second, four on the third ... In the end that doubling process arrives at square sixty-four and he presents the king with a rice debt of more than eighteen quintillion grains of rice – vastly more than the kingdom could produce.

Olen: (*still annoyed*) Thanks for taking the same spoiling approach to my explanations as you always do to my jokes. But actually I was going to tell the story of the person who takes a simple A4 piece of paper and doubles its thickness by folding it in half. By forty-two folds, if you could actually do that, you have a stack that reaches as far as the moon. But these aren't just cute stories. They describe improvement that actually occurs to digital technologies. According to Moore's Law, the number of transistors in an integrated circuit doubles about every two years. That's part of the reason today's lightweight digital devices stream movies while the bigger devices of not so long ago struggled to download simple email messages.

Winston: This sounds to me like a rant about the technologies that made your millions. I don't see what it's got to do with human enhancement.

Olen: (*sounding exasperated*) Can't you see? All we've got to do is get the technologies that make next year's smartphone better than this year's into human heads. The neuroprostheses that are already being introduced into human heads are the way to humanize Moore's Law.

Winston: So we have to replace parts of our biological brains with silicon chips to get the maximum value from these enhancement technologies you've been talking about? This sounds less like a way of humanizing Moore's Law and more like a way to use Moore's Law to dehumanize us. You've always been a lover of sci-fi. You loved the *Terminator* movies. Did you not get any of their messages about the dangers of mixing machine and human? The movies in this franchise involve cyborgs with living human skin over a robotic endoskeleton. I think you might remember the many times in the first two movies when damage jarringly reveals a mechanical interior concealed by human skin.

Olen: I think you're talking about the T-800 series famously played by Arnold Schwarzenegger. And you are getting some of the details of my favourite movie franchise approximately right. But what prevents me from responding to the genocidal T-800 of the original movie, with the very human-friendly versions of Schwarzenegger's T-800 that featured in later movies? Don't you remember later movies in the franchise in which Schwarzenegger's character returns to save humanity, and indeed, goes so far as to arrange its self-termination for our benefit? What a praiseworthy act of cyborg self-sacrifice!

Winston: This does sound too good to be true.

Can we have radically enhanced cognitive powers?

Olen: Do you mind if I take you directly to the most exciting path to radical cognitive enhancement? If we were listening to Eugenie with her marketing of liberal eugenics, we would be hearing about discoveries of genes that influence intelligence. One 2017 study identified twenty-two genes that may be responsible for 5 per cent of the variance in human IQ scores. Eugenie would note that these genes seem particularly active during the brain's development. She might speculate about how tweaking or doubling up on some of these genetic influences might increase human intelligence quite a bit. But I don't think that we have time to wait. Perhaps the genetically enhanced humans of 2200 will understand the destructive potential of the climate crisis. But that's likely to be too late. Here's a suggestion from a dear friend of mine called Ray Kurzweil on how we radically fast-forward cognitive enhancement.

Winston: There's that word "radical" again. This is the Kurzweil of the Singularity? So we are moving from Eugenie's careful attention to scientific discoveries about genes to Kurzweil's love of exponential technological improvement? (*groans*) Back into the realm of superoptimistic science fiction divorced from scientific reality.

Olen: Winston – remember Sophie's lecture on night one about being reasonable? Last night Sophie let you get away with talk of philosophical shit stirring because you managed to persuade her it was a technical term. But please don't dismiss my suggestion until you've heard me out.

Winston: OK Olen, I'm listening. That doesn't mean that I have to enjoy it.

Olen: Ray's crowning novelty is about recognizing that the exponential improvement isn't just about integrated circuits. His Law of Accelerating Returns describes exponential improvement as a feature of all technological change. It's even a feature of evolution. The doubling cycles of evolutionary accelerating returns are more spaced out than the doubling cycles in evolution. In the case of our species the constraint is reproduction. Evolution can spread an advantageous mutation in viruses quite quickly – look at the terrifying efficiency with which the SARS-Cov-2 virus evolved responses to our vaccines. But humans spend years coming of age reproductively and getting the opportunity to pass any advantageous mutations on to the next generation. If we really want to speed things up we will need to replace the evolutionary doublings of biological brains with the digital doublings of neuroprostheses.

Eugenie: So this is supposed to be the difference between Ray's plan and liberal eugenics?

Olen: Only one of them. This is what happens to liberal eugenics when it grows up and gets in touch with digital technology. It's predictable that we are going to begin replacing fallible inefficient biological parts of our brains and bodies with superior digital parts. We will rapidly pass through a stage of being a MOSH, or Mostly Original Substrate Human. This is Ray's term for a human who has very few digital replacement parts or computational implants.

Winston: Can you stop with the "Ray" talk. Is he actually your friend? I strongly suspect that the closest you've come to meeting Kurzweil is watching YouTube clips of him.

Olen: (*now speaking so rapidly and excitedly that he seems barely to have registered Winston's putdown*) Once we see how superior the replacements are we will speedily swap out the biological residue. There are already experiments on neuroprosthetic hippocampi that could replace human hippocampi damaged by Alzheimer's disease. It turns out that damage to the hippocampus is much of the reason for the faulty memories of Alzheimer's patients. Now we need to consider these neuroprostheses in the light of exponential technological change. We won't stop with compensating for the damage done by Alzheimer's. We will create replacements for healthy human hippocampi that harness Moore's Law and other generalizations governing progress in digital technologies. These will grant us superhuman powers of memory.

Sophie: Something tells me you're not finished …

Olen: Now suppose you are really enjoying your new powers of memory. Won't you look at other supposedly healthy parts of your brain and upgrade them with digital tech?

We will become human cyborgs. But the machine parts of our psyches will rapidly replace the biological parts. And yes I've never met Kurzweil *in the flesh*. But I've read his 2005 book *The Singularity is Near* so many times that I feel like I know him. Anyway, the ideas that constitute Kurzweil are increasingly being instantiated digitally.

Winston: *(in a more conciliatory tone)* Wow, so when is this going to happen?

Olen: Soon! Ray … oops sorry … Kurzweil has named 2045 as year of the Singularity. (*Olen flashes up a definition.*)

The Singularity: a "future period during which the pace of technological change will be so rapid, its impact so deep, that human life will be irreversibly transformed."

We can identify the technological singularity as the time on the graph of exponential technological progress when the gradient becomes so steep that it seems to be vertical. Technological advances may seem to come so quickly that they will seem almost instantaneous. Winston and her bioconservative buddies who insist on rejecting technological advances certainly won't be able to keep up then. Fingers crossed there will be MOSH habitats for you Winston. These will be similar to the habitats that we try to maintain for the lowland gorillas. But those of us who have taken advantage of all the new neurotech will have no problem in keeping up. They will understand and enthuse about the destinations that digitally enhanced posthumans are travelling to.

Eugenie: Olen, I'm following you on some of this. But can't you see that this talk about human cyborgs is basically a scam? Why not just fess up that we are going to turn into inhuman machines.

Olen: But we will be human. Swapping out malfunctioning and inefficient biological substrate shouldn't change our values. We will continue to paint pictures and fall in love. We will continue to understand arguments for *The Godfather* being the greatest movie of all time. I always love the episodes of *Star Trek* in which Data demonstrated his fascination for human art forms. Data frequently says he wants to become more human. Think of it this way. If Data is a fully digital being who wants to become more human then it makes sense that we would understand the worth of preserving human values even as we progressively integrate cybernetic components.

Winston: I can't imagine what could possibly go wrong. Actually ... yes I can. I've watched enough dystopian sci-fi to have some sense of what could go wrong. I'm sure the cognitively enhanced beings Olen imagines us becoming will surpass our understanding of how *The Godfather* was made. But one thing that I remember about that movie was that it was all about the trials and tribulations of human beings. We care about the moral decline of Michael Corleone. I understand that you think we'll be able to upload our values into our cybernetically enhanced brains, but how likely is it that we will continue to care about *The Godfather*? I'm betting that if we continue approximately as we are – as MOSHs – then our descendants will still be debating the moral entrapment of Michael Corleone in 2072 and 2172. I find it hard to believe that our cybernetically enhanced descendants will care much about how Michael addressed his moral dilemmas of loyalty to family and respect for universal moral ideals. To put it another way, perhaps they will feel about as emotionally involved in Michael's moral dilemmas as we are in the social dilemmas of some prehuman species.

Olen: (*seems somewhat downcast*) Well perhaps our radically enhanced descendants won't watch *The Godfather* much anymore. I'm a bit sad about that, but only a bit. I'd rather think about the amazing creative experiences of our posthuman descendants.

Will our quest to become a spacefaring species turn us into clouds of nanobots?

Winston: Olen, you're keen to follow Elon into space. Suppose I accept that, if we are to thrive and not just barely survive in space, there's much of our biology that we may need to get rid of. I'm curious to hear more about what you think technology might turn us into. I can see that our evolved biology isn't optimized for space. Olen, you make use of some fantastical thought experiments to present a very optimistic picture of the future effects of enhancement technologies. Are you interested in a thought experiment with the opposite message?

Olen: Sure Professor. Depress us with your forecast of what posthumans optimized for space might look like.

Winston: Unlike you, Olen, I've never pretended to be an expert in digital tech. Suppose we take seriously Musk's plan to turn humanity into a multi-planet, space-faring species. Olen is thrilled about Data's ability to spacewalk without one of those cumbersome spacesuits required to keep his human crewmates on the *Enterprise* alive. I wonder if those future spacefaring posthumans will look anything like us. The character Data was played by Brent Spiner and it's clear that human audiences of the 1990s enjoyed watching him struggle to become more human. But if we were really thinking of the optimal design for a spacefaring posthuman I doubt we'd care much about how endearing they seem to audiences of 1990s humans.

Olen: Now you are the one indulging in crazy tech forecasts! I suppose if I'm allowed to then I can't stop you. At least my future tech thought experiments are designed to be inspiring. I'm saying we can preserve valued aspects of being human into a radically enhanced future. You're saying "I don't think we will." I'm an optimist. There's plenty of data to suggest that optimistic people enjoy better health than pessimists. So, what I'm saying is that even if I don't outlive you by successfully integrating tech into my physiology, my sunny attitude will ensure that you're buried way before me.

Winston: I'm not finished yet, Olen. Here's some evidence that our radically enhanced posthuman descendants will promptly program humanity out. It used to be the case that humans did all of the work extracting valuable ores from deep mineshafts. But mining is dangerous. There's a long history of tragic accidents killing miners. Increasingly we are sending machines underground to do work too dangerous for humans. These are intelligent machines guided by increasingly sophisticated AIs. Guess what. (*Winston displays images of robot miners.*) They don't look much like the human miners they replace. In a scientifically accurate future TV series on the loves and disappointments of mining bots I don't think Brent Spiner will be cast in any of the leading roles. If that's true of machine intelligences optimized for mining then it should also be true for posthuman intelligences optimized for space. It's comparatively easy to send robot probes to Mars. Getting biological humans there is tricky and expensive. But Kurzweil can solve that problem by turning us into robot probes.

Olen: OK Professor. Do you care to venture any guesses?

Winston: These are just speculations. But have you come across Dennis E. Taylor's *Bobiverse* novels? They involve a human Bob Johansson who biologically dies and has his mind uploaded into a computer. Bob's computer mind is placed into a spaceship and heads off into space in search of new homes for humanity and the machines that are *of* humans. Taylor's books are excellent reads, but if I were to venture a guess about the digitally enhanced future I doubt that beings like Bob would manifest any of the interest in unenhanced humans that Bob and his fellow machine intelligences display. If I were placing a bet I suspect that these enhanced spacefaring minds will be too busy exploring the galaxy to be all that worried about finding new homes for the leftovers of the human species that messed planet Earth up.

Olen: OK Professor! So you like the *Bobiverse* novels, but you doubt they are accurate forecasts of our digitally enhanced futures. You seem to disapprove of the Bobiverse future because its spacefaring intelligences preserve some human values. Do you have a pessimistic forecast to offer?

Winston: I'm not going offer a prediction of the future designed to serve my philosophical purposes. But, failing that, can I at least offer you a scenario of how future machine intelligences that are *of* humans *might* evolve. If you were going to design posthumans for space why not clouds of cooperating nanobots? We can upload aspects of our values and psychologies that we especially value into them and then let them work out how best to travel from star to star. A feature of the *Bobiverse* novels is the capacity for these mechanical human descendants to modify every aspect of themselves. How long will these beings preserve the memory chips optimized to store all of Shakespeare's plays and the scholarship on them? In this logically and physically possible scenario, after an initial period, I doubt those posthuman intelligent clouds will be at all interested in the very human dilemmas of the Prince of Denmark in Shakespeare's *Hamlet*. We aren't much interested in the struggles of single cell organisms that evolution turned into us even if Olen tells us we are *of* them. They certainly aren't human. Suppose we give enhancement technologies unrestricted access to our human natures and they optimize us for interstellar travel by turning us into superintelligent clouds of nanobots. These may cover the distance between Sol and Alpha Centauri very efficiently. But you're not going to fool me into thinking that they are human. You may tell me that they are *of* humans. But I speculate that they'll have too much to do to care about the values and interests of the primitive beings from which they originated.

Sophie: I'm not sure about the rest of you, but that's enough speculative sci-fi for me for the time being!

Eugenie: Sophie, I share your complaint about the overdose of digital tech that Olen has subjected us to. I'm going to choose tomorrow's venue and steer the conversation back to the realities of human biology.

Night 5   SENS and radical life extension

Coffee in Curú National Wildlife Refuge, Nicoya, Costa Rica

Sophie: From space to where …? This looks lovely. Eugenie, you brought us here. You do know that we are supposed to be doing philosophy rather than sipping cocktails in whatever tropical holiday destination you've taken us?

Eugenie: Don't worry, our visit has a philosophical purpose. This is not the tropical paradise of getting drunk on the beach. This evening coffee takes place amid the natural splendours of Nicoya, Costa Rica. We will be entertained by families of Capuchin monkeys.

Winston: Those Capuchins are having a great time. I'm almost able to fool myself into thinking they aren't mere Metaverse constructs. But I'm guessing we aren't here to watch the monkeys.

Eugenie: Correct Winston. I chose to have coffee here because Nicoya was listed by Dan Buettner, an American National Geographic Fellow, as one of five Blue Zones – "pockets of people around the world with the highest life expectancy, or with the highest proportions of people who reach age 100." Other locations on Buettner's list are Okinawa, Japan; Sardinia, Italy; Ikaria, Greece; and Loma Linda, California. We know that extreme poverty has a life-shortening effect. But the reverse correlation seems not to obtain. If you look around you won't see

DOI: 10.4324/9781003321613-5

indicators that the longevity of people in Nicoya has come by achieving excessive material wealth.

Winston: So obviously the people of Nicoya have understood something that has eluded wealthier Manhattanites. But I'm guessing that this evening isn't going to be a lecture about the benefits of healthy diets, good friendships, and getting enough sleep.

Eugenie: Correct again, Winston. We are here to consider paths to even more impressive longevity than achieved by the healthy centenarians of Costa Rica. After the extremes of Olen's vision of our collective posthuman future, I'm beginning to doubt technological visions of radically enhancing human capacities. I've come across a vision of a radically enhanced future that would leave us recognizably human. We certainly wouldn't be disturbingly posthuman clouds of nanobots. This is a technological vision of humanity's possible future. But unlike in the sci-fi presentation we got from Olen last night, the tech isn't the star of the show. It plays a strictly subsidiary role. It will ensure that we radically outlive the Blue Zone centenarians by repairing all the damage that just being alive inflicts on the human body. If we can benefit from these technologies, we will remain recognizably human as we celebrate our 501st birthdays.

Radically extended lifespans

Eugenie: One thing I came across in my investigation of the scientific challenges of significantly extending human lifespans is that it's immensely difficult. The twentieth century saw significant extensions of average human life expectancy. But these came through rich world achievements in granting access to clean drinking water, improved healthcare, and better diets. If you are a rich world inhabitant with access to these things, then it's quite difficult to greatly boost your lifespan. The research on Blue Zones may suggest measures capable of adding a few years. There are genetic variants associated with longer lifespans. Perhaps this will help some of us to get closer to that hundred figure. But once you get to 100 there's not much we can currently do to significantly extend lifespans.

Winston: Perhaps there is something we should learn from that.

Eugenie: Winston, you can contentedly go to your grave if you want to. But please don't give up on behalf of the rest of us. The renegade gerontologist Aubrey de Grey has a plan to help those who want them to enjoy millennial lifespans.

Winston: Hmmm. I'll behave. Please tell me more, Eugenie. How is this de Grey character going to make us all immortal?

Eugenie: De Grey isn't so crude as to offer immortality. He accepts that's impossible. An immortal being has a zero probability of death at any point in the future. That clearly can't happen. If the universe ends in a big crunch, then no sentient being that happens to be around then will survive. What he's offering are indefinite lifespans that come with what de Grey calls *negligible senescence*. When we achieve negligible senescence we effectively won't age. We won't celebrate each birthday with the depressing thought that each year brings us closer to death. We will escape the tyranny of the Gompertz Law.

Sophie: I think you'll need to explain that to us. What's this Gompertz Law about?

Eugenie: The Gompertz Law is named for the nineteenth-century British mathematician Benjamin Gompertz. It excludes external causes of death like having a boulder land on you or being blown up in a war. The law focuses instead on the internal causes of death which include parts of your body becoming diseased, or just wearing out. The Gompertz Law states that the probability of not surviving any given year increases exponentially the longer you live. There are different views about the intervals of the Law, but according to one estimate, when you've made it past age 11, your odds of not surviving until your next birthday double every six or seven years.

Sophie: Can you explain the reference to probability in your statement of the Law?

Eugenie: Certainly! It's not so much that you die because you hit a hard upper limit. Rather the probability of dying in any given year increases the longer you live. Jeanne Calment, the French woman who achieved a lifespan of 122 years 164 days, was, on this view an extreme statistical outlier. She must have been very fortunate indeed. Doubtless Calment inherited genetic variants that somewhat boosted her odds and her abstemious lifestyle helped. But Calment reached an age at which the doublings of the Gompertz Law have predictably killed almost everyone. If de Grey manages to make us negligibly senescent we will escape the tyranny of the Gompertz Law. Eventually we'll be taken out by out-of-control buses or by poorly piloted starships. But if we can stop all the internal stuff from going wrong, we should expect, according to one estimate, to live until 1,000.

Sophie: So how is de Grey going to do this?

Eugenie: De Grey thinks we might soon be able to fix all these internal causes of death, meaning that the Gompertz Law will no longer apply to us. Your chances of surviving to your next birthday will be the same in your seventies as in your twenties.

Winston: OK Eugenie, we're all waiting for a story about how to do this that isn't just science fantasy. It's easy to tell stories about waters from magic fountains that grant eternal youth. There seem to be uncountably many diseases that afflict humans. Please don't tell me that de Grey's plan for negligible senescence involves him saying "Step One: Cure every human disease." If so, I'm not buying it.

Can SENS make humans negligibly senescent?

Eugenie: Can someone confirm that there are no sharp objects near Winston. Because that's exactly what I'm going to say. When you telescope down to the level of the cell there are only seven things that go wrong with humans. (*Eugenie summons a display with "Seven Deadly Things" marked on it.*) In the end, we are built out of tiny bits of Lego called human cells. De Grey has counted the seven things that cause cellular death or dysfunction. He calls these the Seven Deadly Things. Winston's looking bored and annoyed, so I will quickly summarize these Deadly Things. There is junk within cells and junk between cells. There are mutations to nuclear DNA – some of which cause cancer. There are mutations to the DNA of mitochondria – the machinery of cells. We lose cells in places we need them and gain them in places we don't. Finally, there are intercellular protein links between cells as we age.

Sophie: That's a lot to take in.

Eugenie: Yes, I'm quite out of breath after running through those! You can refresh your memories by looking up there. Here's a link to a presentation that summarizes the seven deadly things. (*Olen gestures to the floating display: www.gowinglife.com/web-stories/death-by-a-thousand-cuts-the-7-deadly-sins-of-ageing/*) It also contains an image of a youthful but bearded de Grey. Note de Grey's uncanny resemblance to the epically long-lived mythical being Methuselah. The Bible tells us "Thus all the days of Methuselah were nine hundred sixty-nine years; and he died" (*Genesis* 5:27). De Grey is a product of the internet age and he understands the value of marketing. If you're selling a cure for aging, it's important to look the part.

Winston: These seem also to be hallmarks of a digital age scam.

Eugenie: Remember, you promised, Sophie, that you would hear proposals out before you rush to condemn them.

There's more to de Grey than a big beard. The good news is that each of the Seven Deadly Things is fixable. As we live, damage will continue to accumulate, but we can keep on fixing it. De Grey has an analogy involving vintage cars. The more you drive your car the more its parts wear out. But if you were diligent in repairing and replacing its parts then your 1965 VW Beetle could drive every bit as well as it did when it first exited the factory in Wolfsburg. I'm not saying this will be cheap. Humans will be much more expensive to restore to factory-fresh status than VW Beetles.

Winston: That's a cute analogy. But is there any suggestion that de Grey can do for our bodies what Volkswagen engineers can do for '65 Beetles?

Eugenie: De Grey accepts that repairing all of this age-related damage won't be easy. But he's a creative thinker and has loads of suggestions about how to fix each of these Seven Deadly Things. He even has a suggestion about how to cure cancer. He calls it Whole-body Interdiction of Lengthening of Telomeres or WILT. I won't go much into it here. But if it works it will do better than effectively treating cancer when you get it, or reducing your odds of getting cancer. It will make cancer impossible. WILT involves genetically engineering the trillions of cells that comprise human bodies to prevent them from going cancerous in the first place. De Grey wants to then use stem cell technology to replace the cell types that he expects negligibly senescing human bodies to run out of.

Winston: Ahh ... more science fantasy. There must be a catch. How much money does de Grey want for this?

Eugenie: In the early 2000s de Grey expressed the view that SENS could get well underway with the modest figure of one billion US dollars. That sounds like a lot of money. But we spend money on lots of things that are less important than ending human aging. According to the Stockholm International Peace Research Institute, in 2021 total global military spending reached \$2,113 billion. All we need to do is renounce a few tanks, fighter jets, and ICBMs to ensure that the quest to end aging is very well funded indeed.

Sophie: You make it all seem so easy. So why do you think it's not happening?

Eugenie: One problem is that democratic governments find it much easier to spend money on weapons of war than they do on solutions for the problem of aging. Here's an upside to increasing wealth inequality. There are wealthy people today you could easily stump up one billion dollars to end aging. Amazon's Jeff Bezos funds anti-aging research. What we need is for him to come up with the required one billion, rather than a paltry few million, here and there. But funding rejuvenation technology is not restricted to the superrich. If you do have some spare cash why not give it to the foundation founded by de Grey – the Strategies for Engineered Negligible Senescence (SENS) Research Foundation. I'm sure they accept all major credit cards.

Winston: I think we can all agree that far too much money is currently spent on increasingly ingenious ways to kill each other. I agree that an arms race in nuclear submarines is a worse thing to spend money on than SENS. But the question we should ask about that egregious military overspend is whether SENS would be the best way to spend money liberated from the arms race. Investing in green technology seems to me to be morally superior to both.

Sophie: I don't like the suggestion of democratic failure in this. There are certainly billionaires proficient at spouting green platitudes. But how much money are billionaires prepared to spend on green tech compared to colonizing Mars or ending aging?

Winston: I don't want to seem cynical. But too many of today's billionaires are sci-fi fans who grew up watching *Star Trek* and *Star Wars*. They will happily spend their insufficiently taxed billions on plans to make humans a space-faring species or to give us millennial lifespans. But fixing some of the environmental damage caused by industrialization just doesn't seem cool to them.

Sophie: Perhaps Bill Gates is an exception. Winston, you were critical of his 2021 book *How to Avoid a Climate Disaster*. But he does seem prepared to put some of his money where his mouth is. I'm less confident about the aspirations of Elon Musk. Colonizing Mars seems to be mainly about enabling the select few to escape the climate disaster.

Winston: (*glancing away from his Smartphone*) Sure. As you were talking Eugenie I got curious about Aubrey de Grey and his status as a life extension celebrity. We've heard Olen's admiring references to Ray Kurzweil and Elon Musk. I wondered: How did de Grey manage to make the life extension debate seem, in the public imagination at least, to be mainly about him? My internet searches revealed a lot of discussion about de Grey's Seven Deadly Things and how he's going to fix them. It also revealed this. (*Text appears in front of the friends.*)

A heading within the "Aubrey de Grey" Wikipedia page reads "Sexual harassment allegations." This page describes credible claims that the SENS founder abused his position of authority to proposition young women interested in SENS. It describes how SENS had removed de Grey from his position as chief science officer and severed ties with him. (https://en.wikipedia. org/wiki/Aubrey_de_Grey)

Eugenie: (*after a long pause*) That makes me uneasy. I love de Grey's ideas. But I feel disappointed by de Grey the human being. All I can say is that SENS is bigger than one person. Can we focus on the value of de Grey's plans to end aging and not on his questionable conduct as a human being?

Winston: There may be more to it than that. Here's a story run by the journal *Science* that quotes de Grey on his views about women and the war on aging. (*Winston gestures and text appears.*)

those in the aging industry need to use whatever means necessary to fight the war on aging. ... [He] explained ... "It is at the same level of women in World War II sleeping with Nazis to get information. It is a war against aging here. You have to persuade people to give money ... I am the general."

But, Eugenie, I will accept that we're playing according to Sophie's rules. So please go on.

Might SENS actually slow progress toward an enhanced future?

Sophie: Before you continue Eugenie, I have a question about the relationship between your commitment to SENS and your earlier advocacy of eugenics.

Eugenie: I'm listening, Sophie.

Sophie: So the idea behind Galton's original presentation of eugenics was that we manage human reproduction, thereby accelerating evolution's natural way to improve the species. Natural selection tends to preserve the best equipped to survive and reproduce. Galton thought that human experts in heredity could accelerate that natural process by positive measures that would encourage the good-in-birth to increase their procreative efforts and negative measures that would reduce the odds of the bad-in-birth from passing on their substandard hereditary material.

Eugenie: Yes, that's a good quick summary of Galton's views. Remember that my liberal eugenics responded to the moral flaws of that thesis.

Sophie: Yes, but I also seem to remember that there were grounds for doubting that your liberal view was really eugenics at all. Anyway, I worry that if we were to give SENS enough money to fix all the Seven Deadly Things that it might have an effect that is the exact opposite of what Galton hoped to achieve with eugenics. It could lead to a dysgenic deterioration of the human species.

Eugenie: How so?

Sophie: Evolutionary improvement occurs from generation to generation. The fit have improved chances of passing their genes on to the next generation. The unfit have reduced odds. I wonder what the SENS plan to make some of us negligibly senescent will do to that.

Eugenie: De Grey did offer some thoughts about the problem of overpopulation. One way to think about the climate crisis is that it's a problem of too many humans. If humanity's global population were a mere 100,000, I bet we could burn coal to our wasteful hearts' content. But there are now over eight billion of us and our planet can't sustain that much environmental waste. Now suppose that we have a life expectancy of 969 years. The planet will have to support many more humans.

Sophie: That's a different issue from the one I'm getting at. But what's de Grey's solution to the overpopulation problem?

Eugenie: Please remember that I'm happier focusing on the scientific details of SENS than on the foibles of de Grey the human being. But de Grey's solution is that those who accept the indefinite lifespans of negligible senescence are subject to a moral obligation to not have children. De Grey himself has chosen to remain childless to morally prepare for his Methuselah-like lifespan. In the future society de Grey imagines there will be two kinds of people, those who select the pleasures of negligible senescence and those who select the pleasures of having children. But it will be morally wrong to choose both.

Winston: (*clearly getting angry*) That all sounds very nice, in principle. But I wonder how it will go in practice. How many billionaire Methuselahs will accept a moral requirement that they remain childless? Call me a cynic, but I suspect there is a hint in the many billionaires who refuse to meet their moral obligations to pay fair amounts of tax. One of the main deterrents for poorer people having children is the escalating costs of raising them. Being a working parent is much more challenging today than it was fifty years ago. But if you have the financial resources to easily pay for childcare and the most elite schools then why not spend the healthy years that SENS might give you adding to your brood. Will we see competitions among billionaires to see who can tally the most children? There are already competitions among billionaires whose interest in art came only once they had achieved superrich status to own the most valuable modern artworks.

Eugenie: Trust you to always lower the tone, Winston! Your idea of a competition among negligibly senescent billionaires to have the most babies seems like it might make for an interesting dystopian sci-fi movie but I'm afraid it's a bit mad as a prediction of the effects of SENS.

Winston: This is just a story about something that could happen. As far as I can see my negligibly senescent billionaire baby competition thought experiment violates no laws of logic or physics. It could happen! I think it can be useful to consider such stories as we enter an essentially uncertain future. Wouldn't considering it insure us against it happening. I'm pretty sure my house won't burn down but I nevertheless insure it. This is more than just a thought experiment. At last count, Olen's hero Elon Musk has ten children. How can we be sure that the negligibly senescent wealthy people of the future won't be more like fecund Musk than childless de Grey?

Sophie: That's not the issue I want to raise. There seems to be a tension between Galton's plan of speeding up human evolution and the SENS plan of keeping people alive for as long as money will permit. I've already spoken about my use of a digital technology – my insulin pump – to treat my diabetes. I indulged in a conjecture about a possible future pump that outperforms biologically normal human pancreases. Here's a different philosophical use of my diabetes. I haven't seen reports of German diabetics being euthanized in the Nazi T4 eugenics programme. But there is a significant inherited contribution to Type 1 diabetes. I remember when my doctor diagnosed me and put me on insulin, he speculated about the dysgenic consequences of insulin injections. That didn't make me feel great. But it is true that without them I would have died and my faulty DNA would have been eradicated from the human gene pool. Eugenicists might view my death before achieving reproductive age as improving the human species.

Eugenie: Where are you going with this Sophie? I can certainly understand why you'd be angry at your callous doctor.

Sophie: Suppose Galton would have relegated me to the class of the dysgenic – my diabetes makes me bad-in-birth. By good luck I have access to the best rejuvenation technologies. I also take advantage of the youthful state that SENS has secured for me to have many children slowing down the evolutionary path of improvement that Galton hoped to accelerate.

Olen: Sorry Sophie but I'm not sure what we are supposed to make of these speculations in a philosophical discussion about human enhancement.

Sophie: Perhaps they are just a way to level the philosophical playing field. Olen, you spent these past evenings selling the beautiful futures that enhancement technologies could engineer for humanity. Sometimes you seem unjustifiably certain about them. But under cross-examination you have thankfully become less confident. I can't be certain about my story in which I use SENS to have hundreds of diabetic children. I'm guessing that diabetes is easier to fix than cancer. But remember that there are no guarantees about the future. Pro-enhancement philosophers love the stories in which the promises of enhancement tech are fully realized. It's good for philosophers to also listen to stories in which enhancement technologies fail of to live up to their inventors' aspirations.

Do we need to escape human biology if we are going to live to be 969?

Olen: I don't want to put even more strain on Eugenie's and my pro-enhancement alliance, but there is one issue that I have with SENS. It really doesn't go far enough. It's all very well to have a plan to fix all of the Seven Deadly Things. But some of them seem very difficult to fix indeed – much more difficult than de Grey makes out. You mentioned WILT, Eugenie. We've already discussed Siddhartha Mukherjee's 2010 book *The Emperor of all Maladies*. In his history, the imminent end of cancer has been frequently forecast. We got many ingenious therapies. I'd be happier to receive a cancer diagnosis today than when President Nixon declared war on the disease. But none of the predicted cures for cancer arrived. De Grey is clearly a smart guy with some interesting speculations about cancer. But smart people have long been promising to cure cancer and not delivering. There is a great example in which the authoritative *New York Times* carried a story by one of its science journalists reporting a claim by the Nobel laureate James Watson that cancer would be cured within two years. That story ran in 1998. When it comes to promised cures for cancer we are easily fooled. Reading Mukherjee's book has only increased my doubts about de Grey's breezy plan to cure cancer by making it impossible for humans to get it.

Sophie: Given what you've been saying about progress in digital technologies, it's interesting to hear you playing the role of enhancement tech sceptic.

Olen: Yes Sophie. But my scepticism is really just about an approach that anchors our destinies too closely to the details of our biology. I doubt we'll ever see de Grey's predicted WILT cure for cancer. And Mukherjee is smart enough to see why. According to him, cancer is built into our natures as biological beings.

Eugenie: Wow! This is a very different Olen. So now you're joining Winston in the bioconservative camp?

Olen: Perish the thought! Mine is a complaint about half-measures in the Age of Human Enhancement. The best way to make cancer impossible is for humanity to forsake its biology. Machines don't get metastases! And this is likely to apply to the challenges posed by the other Seven Deadly Things. We need to retire our antiquated biological tech replacing it as quickly as we can with digital tech.

Eugenie: So what you're saying is – give up on fixing our evolved biologies billions of years in the making? I think I can see where you're coming from. Businesses sometimes get too attached to their legacy technologies when they should be scrapping them and starting over. But this is where you and I part company, Olen. We may be broadly in favour of human enhancement. But I'm not happy with Kurzweil's plan to delete the "biological human" from "human enhancement." I'd rather stick with the SENS plan to prepare and cautiously update humanity's evolved legacy tech.

Olen: Thanks Eugenie. I'm optimistic that history will bear me out. Kurzweil has an amazing record as a forecaster of tech developments. It's not for nothing that he has been hailed as the "Nostradamus for the Digital Age." His accolades for successful forecasting don't come from the mystical resources of Nostradamus but from application of the Law of Accelerating Returns. Many of Kurzweil's forecasts that seemed mad at the time he made them – such as victories of computers over the best human chess players and massive increases in usage of the internet – turned out to be true. I know that Winston enjoys pouring scorn on anyone who thinks differently, but if I was a betting person, I'd be more convinced by Google's 2012 hiring of Kurzweil. There's a company with a demonstrated capacity to make money out of the future direction of digital tech.

The choice between moderate and radical enhancement

Eugenie: I think it's time for me to speak up more forcefully here. (*Eugenie turns to address all of her friends.*) Up until recently I've been very happy to join Olen as a member of team enhancement. It's good to have friends in a serious philosophical debate just as it's good to have allies in a fistfight. But I have to confess that all of Olen's ecstatic advocacy of our enhanced future is making me dizzy. Some of Winston's objections are beginning to make sense to me.

Winston: Finally!

Eugenie: Not so fast, Winston. I am an advocate of human enhancement. It's good that we take advantage of some of the possibilities opened up by enhancement technologies. Moreover, I accept that in the long run we might end up changing quite a lot. But your thought experiment in which we might be expected to celebrate becoming clouds of nanobots so long as that makes interstellar travel a bit easier worries me. Perhaps those clouds will be *of* humans. But the clouds don't carry forward the things that I value about being human. I can accept that over the long run we may become very different kinds of beings. But that doesn't mean that the human future should be dictated by the timetable of exponential progress.

Olen: This sounds like betrayal of the very idea of enhancement to me. I'm saying human enhancement is good so

I want as much of it as I can get. What are you saying? Human enhancement is maybe good but you shouldn't want too much of it?

Eugenie: Unlike you, Olen, I accept that I will eventually die. I certainly don't want to die tomorrow. Perhaps in the *very* distant future we will become space-faring clouds of nanobots. But I don't want to personally become that. And I don't want my child to be that. What would the clouds of nanobots be like to cuddle? I would find it hard to imagine how the kinds of loving relationship between mother and daughter that are part of what I celebrate about being human could survive into a future that has taken the path Olen is counselling. I don't think I could love a child who has become a space-faring cloud of nanobots even if Olen assures me it's not only *of* humanity but my direct descendant.

Sophie: OK Eugenie. I think my toothache is back. (*Sophie rubs her jaw.*) That may be making me more amenable to Olen's marketing of radical enhancement as a way to end nature's use of dental pain to tyrannize us. So how is your use of enhancement technologies really different from what Olen is proposing?

Eugenie: I accept that enhancement technologies will and should change us. Suppose a historian of the thirtieth century were to look back on a time when we've been able to apply enhancement technologies, including gene editing, to ourselves, they would identify the Age of Human Enhancement as a time of accelerated change in the human species and what it means to be human. But there is an important difference between the radical enhancement that Olen is selling and moderate enhancement which improves its subjects within or just beyond the normal biological range of humans. I understand that if we keep on adding moderate enhancements the net effect will be radical enhancement. But I also understand that the eventual effect of all of the damage that my body gradually accumulates over time is death. Unlike Olen I'm fine with the thought that I will eventually die. I am hoping that some of SENS's rejuvenation technologies will work. I accept that some may not. This may mean that I don't live quite as long as Methuselah. But I'm fine with this, so long as I can remain recognizably human. I refuse to do as Olen recommends and upload myself on to one of his computers.

Sophie: So unlike Olen you don't fear death?

Eugenie: I'm fine about eventually dying. I prefer to get there gradually and incrementally rather than all at once, ASAP. I feel the same about enhancing too quickly. I fear that it will terminate my connections with other humans and ruin my enjoyment of distinctively human values and pleasures.

Olen: (*voice raising angrily*) Eugenie, I hereby terminate our pro-enhancement alliance! Honestly, I've never heard such nonsense. We are trying to have a rational conversation about human enhancement and here you are comparing enhancing yourself with dying.

Eugenie: Actually, Olen, I think you're getting a bit forgetful there – you already terminated our philosophical alliance. Does this explain your interest in rejuvenation tech? My comparison of enhancement with death is an analogy. There clearly are differences. But differences don't prevent an analogy from being philosophically useful.

Winston: Perhaps you can give us an example?

Sophie: I think I will duck out of this philosophical fight between advocates of enhancement. I just made a booking with my dentist.

Eugenie: See you tomorrow evening, Sophie. It looks like I will temporarily be taking on your role as philosophical supervisor. Winston, here's a good example of how a philosophical analogy can work. Judith Jarvis Thomson famously compared the moral relationship between you and a famous violinist who is attached to you without your consent and who will die if you disconnect, and that between a pregnant woman and her foetus. She argues that if you are morally entitled to detach from a violinist, a pregnant woman is entitled to terminate the relationship of dependence between herself and her foetus. This is a philosophically informative analogy even if there clearly are differences between sick violinists and foetuses. My comparison of enhancement with the process of dying is informative even if dying and being enhanced are clearly different processes.

Olen: I can see the philosophical value of well-chosen analogies, but dying and being enhanced seem like diametrically opposed processes to me.

Eugenie: Here's where I want to hear from Winston. Olen has convinced me that exponentially improving digital technologies could radically transform us and our descendants. I fear that if radically enhancing digital technologies turned my child – or my future selves – into a cloud of cooperating space-faring nanobots I might have difficulty relating to its experiences. Would it even have experiences? I might view the application of enhancement technologies that has this effect as coming close to killing me. If you applied those enhancement technologies to my child I might have difficulty feeling the very human emotion of love for them. Sophie was feeling dizzy with all of her painkillers. I think I'm feeling a bit dizzy with all this sci-fi. I'm keen to hear more from Winston about how this philosophy by sci-fi could apply to choices that we may make soon about enhancing ourselves and our kids.

Winston: Thanks for your generous expression of philosophical bipartisanship on this issue. I'm grateful for the way a member of team enhancement can reach across the aisle to listen to the view of someone previously derided as a bioconservative. I have to confess that I've been doing a great deal of reading in the Great Library to get clarity on the broader human effects of enhancement. My survey is taking me on a fascinating tour of readings beyond the Library's philosophy shelves. I propose that we dedicate an entire evening to exploration of these issues. In the meantime I have a question for Eugenie.

Eugenie: I'm all ears.

Why advocates of moderate enhancement might prefer gene editing to enhancement by digital tech

Winston: Suppose we do manage to make this distinction between radical and moderate enhancement philosophically principled. How would you apply it to the various enhancement technologies that Olen has been marketing?

Eugenie: I agree that it's not going to be easy to draw this line and make it philosophically principled. Philosophically speaking Olen's job is easy. He seems up for any and all enhancements. To paraphrase him, the more the merrier. The appeal to him of digital technologies as enhancement technologies is that the exponential pattern of improvement seems capable of delivering very powerful enhancement techs very soon. We've heard that for Olen there's no "enough" with human enhancement. But we mustn't forget that we are talking about *human* enhancement. Philosophers have struggled for millennia to answer questions about what it means to be human and what's important about being human. This distinctively philosophical dispute isn't like many disputes in science that we expect to find definitive answers to. For as long as there are humans there will be intense debates about what it means to be human and what are the truly important things about being human. Aristotle's writings on human reproduction are not required readings in today's biology courses. But his writings on what it means to be human and what's involved in being a

	good human are keenly enjoyed in today's philosophy courses.
Olen:	Sophie was the one we were looking to for philosophical clarification. Now that she's out of commission with toothache you seem determined to make things more complicated, Eugenie.
Eugenie:	All I'm saying is that, in philosophy at least, complex problems deserve complex solutions. I think it was Sophie who quoted Einstein – "Everything should be made as simple as possible, but not simpler." Humans are complex and Olen's answer to the question of human enhancement is too simple.
Olen:	OK Eugenie. I'm looking forward – or not! – to Eugenie's explanation of why enhancing is a bit like dying. I will need to bear in mind Sophie's warning about being civil. My question about what you've just said is – how does your advocacy of moderate enhancement apply to the enhancement techs we've been discussing?
Eugenie:	Thank you Olen. Our investigation of enhancement began with a discussion of Galton and his morally misguided plan to enhance our species by managing human reproduction. I presented liberal eugenics as a response to the injustices of authoritarian eugenics. Olen, I got the impression that you viewed its focus on human hereditary material as a tad retro.
Olen:	Only because we have a collection of exponentially improving digital technologies that are guaranteed to pick up the pace of human enhancement. We don't have to mess around with adding additional copies of genes that we believe to be important in the development of the human brain. We don't have to limit ourselves to upregulating the expression of genes that make our brain tissue more connective.
Eugenie:	I'm thinking that if we can find a way to make moderate enhancement philosophically principled that the limitations of genetic enhancement might be an asset

rather than a disadvantage. We had the lecture from Olen about the exciting surprises delivered by exponentially improving digital technologies. Today's computers are not just a bit more powerful than those of ten years ago, they are hugely more powerful. My reading in the Great Library alerted me to a distinction made by mathematicians when discussing change over time. Olen gave us a very instructive tutorial on exponential change. There is a difference between that and arithmetic change. In an arithmetic sequence change occurs by a fixed amount. We can contrast the exponential doubling sequence with the arithmetic plus two sequence. Suppose that introducing additional copies of genes that influence the development of the brain produced arithmetic improvement. Its products are more likely to be acknowledged by the unenhanced among us as fellow humans. Consider someone who is a bit smarter than the rest of us because she has brain tissue that's more connective. If that individual was my daughter I might accept that she is more intelligent than me but I would have no difficulty in acknowledging her as human.

Winston: We are going to need an example to illustrate how this could happen, Eugenie.

Eugenie: Why not! Here's a possible application of gene editing to human beings. The NR2B gene is known to be active during the development of parts of the mammalian brain linked with learning. In an experiment in the 1990s geneticists added an extra copy of NR2B to a mouse embryo. The resulting "Doogie" mouse outperformed unmodified mice in tests of memory and learning. Humans aren't mice but mice and humans are both mammals. When news of the Doogie mouse was broken people speculated about the effects on humans of adding an extra NR2B gene to a human embryo.

Winston: I do hope you're not advocating this, Eugenie.

Eugenie: No, for the time being I'm happy to advance it as a thought experiment. What would we say about a human with an additional copy of NR2B who enjoyed the same advantages over their peers as Doogie mice do over normal mice? I think this enhanced Doogie human is much more easily recognized as human than are the radically enhanced beings that could result from the exponentially improving digital technologies that so excite Olen.

Winston: I'm glad you aren't advocating actually inserting extra copies of NR2B into human embryos. I have come across a report that enhanced memories and learning seem to have come at a cost for Doogie mice. These enhanced mice seemed to suffer from something like post-traumatic stress disorder. In one experiment Doogie mice and controls were subjected to mild electric shocks when they neared landmarks in their environment. This may seem like an example of scientists torturing their nonhuman experimental subjects just because they can. But there were interesting lessons learned from this. The electric shocks ceased and the normal mice gradually lost their fear. But the Doogie mice didn't. They seemed to be stuck with mouse PTSD.

Eugenie: This is why I'm happy for this to be nothing more than a useful philosophical thought experiment until we confirm that it's safe. We will want to sort out that PTSD issue before any human child is born with this. But my belief in scientific and technological progress suggests to me that we will solve it. When we do sort out the Doogie mice PTSD issue I'm confident we'll get the enhanced human intellects without the angst. When we do we will have happy children who are smarter than us, but still lovably human.

Winston: That's fine, Eugenie. But I think there's something a bit fishy about the way advocates of enhancement use thought experiments. I think we will need to address this issue later.

Eugenie: Perhaps when Sophie is back.

Olen: I have a question about your moderate view, Eugenie. So your technologically retro approach to enhancement has an advantage for those who like you are a bit timid about our enhanced future. Unlike you I'm excited about all of the possibilities opened up by a future in which we use technology to bust out of the straightjacket of our evolved humanity. I don't see what's wrong with our radically enhanced descendants looking back on our current version of humanity with some nostalgia but also with a sense that they don't want to go back. But I have another question for you, Eugenie.

Eugenie: Go on.

Olen: You don't have children yet. But I'm disappointed to hear that if you were to radically enhance your child you might struggle to love them. Are your maternal instincts so shallow that you could love a child who was a bit smarter than you but you'd struggle to love one that was much, much smarter than you?

Eugenie: All I'm saying is that we are yet to conduct that experiment on the power of human maternal or paternal love. Before we apply enhancement technologies to the next generation in the unrestricted way you seem to be urging, Olen, let's not lazily assume that love can conquer any intergenerational barrier created by enhancement technologies.

Winston: Can you come up with an example to bolster your case? I understand that it won't be an actual case. We don't have data from parents who've radically enhanced their children. Can you use any imaginary case, say from fiction, that might help us to understand why too much enhancement might create a barrier between parent and child? There doesn't have to be an exact fit. But since we are entering philosophically uncharted waters here, we need all the help we can get.

Eugenie: Actually, I do have a fictional case that, though not an exact fit, may help. It's the 1957 sci-fi novel *The Midwich Cuckoos* written by British author John Wyndam. It was turned into a TV series that played in 2022. In the novel a mysterious event renders all of the inhabitants of a British village unconscious. When they awake all of the women find that they are pregnant. The kids are born and seem normal, apart from their golden eyes and silvery skin. All of them have blonde hair. We then learn that they have unusual abilities such as telekinesis, telepathy, and mind control. The most arresting passages in *The Midwich Cuckoos* involve their parents struggling to love their children, even as the children increasingly perceive mum and dad as potential existential threats demanding lethal responses.

Olen: Sorry but this is not a useful analogy. *The Midwich Cuckoo* kids are extraterrestrials!

Eugenie: It's clearly not a perfect analogy. But as I said before, we need cases like these to get a fix on what parenting a child with superhuman capacities might be like. We can't just suppose that the bond between parent and radically enhanced child will be no different from the bond between parent and unenhanced child.

Winston: Excellent. I'm very much looking forward to later discussions. I'm confident I can convince you, and win Eugenie over to my side.

Eugenie: I doubt that very much.

Winston: I think it's time to set the agenda for tomorrow evening's discussion. I'm very much looking forward to Sophie's return.

Olen: So, we've looked at cognitive enhancement and life extension. There are two other topics that I'd like to discuss tomorrow. I predict that then you'll have a full picture of the joys of human enhancement and will join with me in endorsing the purest commitment to improving humanity that is radical human enhancement.

Winston: So what are tomorrow's topics, Olen?

Olen: Well, your depressing negativity about enhancement technologies is affecting even my effervescent optimism, Winston. I want to look at technologies that will make us all much happier. But just to prove that I am not a blinkered optimist, I want also to introduce you to moral bioenhancement, which is a way to ensure that we and our descendants make the morally best use of these powerful techs.

Winston: I'm predicting that this will *not* boost my philosophically appropriate low mood.

Night 6 Enhanced moods and morality

Coffee in the World State city of London in 632 AF (After Ford)

Winston: So where on Earth are we now?

Olen: Again, I have to sort out your "on Earth" confusion. We are still physically in the Filthy Spoon Café. You do remember coming here, don't you? But we are virtually in the London of Aldous Huxley's dystopian 1932 novel *Brave New World*. As to when we are: In Huxley's novel there is a new calendar. Huxley's imagined society has followed the lead of Henry Ford, the pioneer of mass production. The architects of Huxley's society have used those principles to create a state of plenty for all. The novel takes place in 632 After Ford (AF). That translates to 2540 CE on our Gregorian calendar.

Sophie: So why are we here?

Olen: Huxley's World State has solved the problem of unhappiness. People boost their happiness by taking a drug called Soma. It also serves a valuable social purpose, ensuring the contentment of the World State's citizenry. Soma turns out to be a very potent happiness drug. Here's Huxley's pitch – "there is always soma, delicious soma, half a gramme for a half-holiday, a gramme for a week-end, two grammes for a trip to the gorgeous East, three for a dark eternity on the moon." As Huxley presents Soma, it has "All the advantages of Christianity and alcohol; none of their defects."

DOI: 10.4324/9781003321613-6

Sophie: (*arranges for her avatar to manifest extreme confusion*) Hang on ... Like you, Olen, and I suspect Winston and Eugenie, I studied *Brave New World* at school. You mentioned the word yourself. Huxley's novel is a *dystopia*! You seem to be thoughtlessly repurposing it to market drugs that boost our moods. When I read the novel I got Huxley's message about the shallowness of human existence in a society that commits itself to enhancing its citizens' affects. What's next? Will you be using George Orwell's *1984* to market a totalitarian state that takes every opportunity to lie to its citizens?

Olen: I agree that Huxley intended his London of 632 AF to be a dystopia. But sometimes an inventive mind like Huxley's can be wrong about the true meaning of a creative vision. I take the lead of the Canadian philosopher Mark Walker. In his 2013 book *Happy-People-Pills For All*, Walker defuses Huxley's anxieties about his dystopia and turns it into a positive vision for society. If we have the pharmacological means to make people happier, surely we should use them. If the future offers even more powerful means of *affective enhancement*, then we should celebrate their imminent arrival.

Winston: So you're calling this plan to give us all Soma, affective enhancement, affective because it focuses on our moods, feelings, and attitudes. Affective enhancement aims to create more joy, interest, and contentment. This sounds like more tech-utopian storytelling. You won't be surprised to hear that I want to continue to read *Brave New World* as a dystopia.

Olen: No, I'm not surprised. But you shouldn't be surprised that I don't want to stop at Soma. My commitment to affective enhancement endorses whatever happiness pill, gene edit, or cybernetic add-on systematically enhances our moods. When it comes to affective enhancement the more the merrier.

Winston: What I'm waiting for is some kind of response to my concern that something might go wrong with the application of all of these increasingly powerful enhancement technologies to our fragile and increasingly vulnerable human natures. Almost a century after the technological wonder of the A-bomb we remain reluctant to question our unthinking commitment to increasingly technological futures. Do you have anything to say in response to the question: How might this go wrong?

Olen: Unlike you I'm an optimist. We simply aren't doomed to repeat yesteryear's worst mistakes. But I have put some thought into ensuring that enhancement technologies will be put to morally good purposes. Winston, all of your fears will be addressed by moral bioenhancement. We will soon have access to pharmaceuticals that morally improve us, helping us to make good uses of exponentially improving technologies. We can dream of an imminent future in which moral enhancement comes from gene edits and cybernetic implants. Why not a future morally perfect humanity?

Happy-people-pills for all?

Sophie: So affective enhancement? Given the way our discussions about enhancement technologies have gone on previous evenings, I'm guessing that we will hear Olen rushing to use digital technologies to radically enhance our affective states. How are we going to bring eternal bliss to humanity?

Winston: Hmm ... I had thought that promises of eternal bliss were the province of the Good Book, or good books plural.

Eugenie: Before Olen gets in here can I offer a very reasonable and moderate pathway to a happier humanity. Walker's 2013 book *Happy-People-Pills For All* advances arguments that are not founded in speculations about future digital techs. He grounds his proposal in scientifically well-supported studies about genetic contributors to happiness. Walker is especially interested in people who are naturally hyperthymic. Members of this fortunate group have more frequent positive moods and emotions than the rest of us. Even if the term "hyperthymic" is new to you, you all know hyperthymic people. They are people who are naturally upbeat who seem resistant to low moods even when life turns against them. Tragic things happen to hyperthymic people, and they certainly do not respond to the death of a loved one with joy. But they find themselves able to respond appropriately to tragedy and then able to move forward with optimism. Winston, you are *not* hyperthymic. You are dysthymic – inclined to low moods. This is certainly not clinical depression. But there is surely a link. There are different estimates about how many among us are hyperthymic but we know that it's a real category. The interest of medical establishment in the very unhappy and how to treat them means that the hyperthymic haven't received the attention from scientists that they deserve.

Winston: I have a view about why that is. Dysthymia attracts more attention from scientists than hyperthymia because there's such a big global market for antidepressants. I wonder if the real goal of Walker's book is to point the way to even greater profits from happiness pills taken by people who would never be diagnosed with depression. Peter Kramer's 1993 book *Listening to Prozac: A Psychiatrist Explores Antidepressant Drugs and the Remaking of the Self* was a step in that direction. Kramer pushed for "cosmetic pharmacology" in which many normally happy people would be taking Prozac to be even happier. It turned out that Prozac and other selective serotonin reuptake inhibitors (SSRIs) have side effects that non-depressed people don't like. So Walker's happiness pills will need to do better than this.

Sophie: So what is Walker's proposal?

Eugenie: Walker begins with studies on genetic differences between the hyperthymic and the rest of us. He proposes to make use of that work to make more of us hyperthymic. In short, he calls for the development of happy pills, pharmaceuticals that supply the brains of the non-hyperthymic with the chemicals that the genes of the hyperthymic naturally supply to their brains.

Winston: So not Prozac then?

Eugenie: That's right, Winston. Some future drug that makes the brains of the non-hyperthymic like the brains of the hyperthymic. So there's no reason to think that the sexual dysfunction that is a common side effect of SSRIs will carry over to Walker's happy pills.

Winston: I'd like to register a distinctively non-hyperthymic objection, here. You guys have known me for many years now. I've always been a tad downbeat. And yes, I have suffered depression. I'm not depressed now. But as you might predict from my contributions to these discussions I probably didn't inherit the genetic variants that interest Walker. But I'm actually fine with that. Moreover I credit my downbeat mood with my productivity as a young academic. Did you know that I just won a prize for emerging historians with especially impressive research records? Could I have done that if I'd been blissed out on the drugs that Walker wants to prescribe me?

Eugenie: First Winston, Walker is a liberal. He doesn't want to force you to be happier. If you insist on your right to be unhappy he's not going to compel you. Rather, he's calling for society to support the development of pharmaceuticals that could be available to the rest of us. Consider someone who has a persistently low mood but doesn't celebrate being a misery guts in the way you do.

Winston: Thanks for not forcibly drugging me! But I'm still not convinced that Walker's happy pills are things that society should spend money on. We shouldn't think that there is an infinite supply of money to spend on anything that some philosopher thinks might be fun to research. I'm not sure if you've heard of our current big problem of anthropogenic climate change ... (*Winston's avatar adopts a mocking aspect.*) Even if Walker convinces me it might be fun to be happier I wouldn't want to invest money on happy-pill research before we've worked out how to sequester this atmospheric carbon our civilization has created.

Eugenie: Walker argues that the two projects may be linked. He cites evidence for a link between higher levels of happiness and pro-social behaviour. In this tainted age pro-social behaviour could easily manifest as positive action on the climate.

Winston: What about the complaint expressed by Huxley's character, John the Savage. John rejects Soma with the line "But I don't want comfort. I want God, I want poetry, I want real danger, I want freedom, I want goodness. I want sin." He prefers these to the bland contentment offered by Soma.

Eugenie: Walker has an answer to that too. He challenges Huxley's notion that we must choose between the happy state offered by Soma and achievement. Walker cites evidence that positive moods and emotions lead to greater levels of achievement. So there's reason to believe that making more of us hyperthymic will lead to more and better poetry.

Winston: I'm still with John the Savage.

Eugenie: Can I quote *Brave New World* back at you just to make sure you are aware of what you are rejecting? In Huxley's novel John is asked whether he really wants to claim: (*Text appears.*)

the right to grow old and ugly and impotent; the right to have syphilis and cancer; the right to have too little to eat; the right to be lousy; the right to live in constant apprehension of what may happen tomorrow; the right to catch typhoid; the right to be tortured by unspeakable pains of every kind.

John responds "I claim them all." Are you that daring, Winston?

Winston: I don't think I have to claim them all. I claim some of them. I want to use technology to fix problems but in a way that leaves my humanity intact. Of the items on that list I claim the right to grow old and ugly and impotent and the right to live in constant apprehension of what may happen tomorrow. I also claim the right to be unhappy. I will use technology to fix the rest.

Can we achieve radically enhanced happiness?

Sophie: I note that Eugenie is the member of team enhancement who has taken the lead in arguing for affective enhancement. This seems to suggest that this goal fits better with her plan to moderately enhance human beings. Nature already creates hyperthymic people. Having a somewhat lower mood would not be classified as a disease state by a doctor. Taking one of Walker's imagined happy pills is therefore an enhancement rather than a therapy. But making Winston hyperthymic wouldn't produce in him emotional states that are far beyond what is possible for any biologically normal human. It wouldn't be a case of radical affective enhancement. Are there any thoughts on what might count as radical enhancement of human moods?

Olen: The transhumanist philosopher Nick Bostrom concedes that it is "difficult to say what would constitute a 'posthuman' level of emotional capacity." But he seems generally optimistic that we could become "posthumanly happy beings." According to Bostrom, some mental gymnastics may be required to begin to conceive of posthuman happiness. Imagining that state will require us to "abstract from contingent features of the human psyche." He advances the conjecture that experiences "that would consume us" could "be merely 'spicy' to a posthuman mind." Bostrom offers a "parallel case" from normal human psychological development to suggest the possibility of posthuman happiness. (*Olen gestures and text appears.*)

The experience of romantic love is something that many of us place a high value on. Yet it is notoriously difficult for a child or a prepubescent teenager to comprehend the meaning of romantic love or why adults should make so much fuss about this experience. Perhaps we are all currently in the situation of children relative to the emotions, passions, and mental states that posthuman beings could experience. We may have no idea of what we are missing out on until we attain posthuman emotional capacities.

Winston: That's an interesting proposition for those offered radical enhancement of their affective states. Effectively he's saying that we may not able to know what it's like until we've submitted to it.

Olen: But Bostrom's example of romantic love suggests that once we get there we'll like it.

Winston: There's something fishy about that reasoning. I propose that we make it a topic for tomorrow evening.

Can we control exponentially improving digital technologies?

Winston: We've heard Eugenie's plea for moderation. But I agree with you, Olen, that yours is the clearest and most emphatic statement of the enhancement ideal.

Olen: Why thank you, Winston, an unexpected compliment.

Winston: OK. But suppose we accept your story about radical human enhancement. Your pitch seemed to be largely premised on exponential technological progress and the enhancements it may offer. This is all supposed to arrive much sooner than we expect, if I understand the message of your paper-folding example. Isn't this all a bit naïve about humanity's capacity to correctly use powerful technologies? I hope I don't have to remind you of the dropping of nuclear bombs on Hiroshima and Nagasaki. Those deaths were consequences of the misuse of powerful technology by unenhanced humans. I wonder and worry about the moral magnitude of the errors of our cybernetically enhanced descendants or future selves.

Olen: I want to register my increasing annoyance at all of the random examples you're throwing around, Winston. We are trying to have a conversation about the potential benefits or harms of radical enhancement. Now you're talking about dropping A-bombs on Japanese cities in World War II. How could this possibly be relevant to our discussion? You're seeming like a hack politician conducting a smear campaign. Neuroprostheses designed to radically enhance cognitive performance and nukes designed to kill people are entirely distinct technologies. Developing one doesn't automatically give you the other. It is absurd to say that radically enhancing our cognitive abilities and extending our lifespans places the Hiroshima nuke in our hands.

Winston: (*adopting an offended tone*) Olen, there is philosophical method in what you interpret as my rhetorical madness. We are trying to get a philosophical fix on the morality of radically enhancing humans. Sophie strongly advised us to not be overconfident in our assertions. If we are seeking advice about an essentially uncertain future in which we apply technology to ourselves then we must consider a variety of examples that potentially reveal otherwise overlooked aspects of applying technology to our human natures. The nuclear bomb analogy serves to highlight what can go wrong if we misuse powerful technology.

Olen: That all presumes that dropping nuclear bombs on Japan to bring a hideously destructive war to an end was morally wrong.

Winston: Quite! I'm convinced it was. But there are many examples of the misuse of technology more obviously germane to our discussion. Kurzweil wants us to progressively replace part of our biological brains with digital enhancements. There's nothing about the way human-machines of the future are built that means that the couldn't preserve our values and continue to enjoy the fiction of Jane Austen. I understand that possibility doesn't violate the laws of logic or physics. But there is another approach to the future that advises caution about new technologies.

Olen: So what approach to the future of enhancement technologies do you recommend?

Winston: If we're exercising prudence about these powerful technologies and all of their unknowable consequences shouldn't we be risk averse? The *Terminator* movies suggest that there's nothing about the architecture of the T-800 that means it couldn't be programmed to not only save Sarah Connor rather than killing her but also to enjoy reading Jane Austen. But doesn't that overlook the message of the franchise which is to ask what could possibly go wrong.

Olen: That's always your first question, isn't it, Winston. Why not join Kurzweil and start with: What could go right? But I think I understand your concerns. Don't worry, I do have a fix.

Winston: More sci-fi wonder tech?

Olen: Not at all. Many of sci-fi's AIs are evil. We shouldn't rule out this possibility. Evil AIs originate from human designers making morally bad choices. Would news that there is a fix for humanity's moral errors that's already on its way address your concerns? We need moral bioenhancement. (*Olen gestures and a definition appears.*) Here's how the Swedish philosopher Ingmar Persson and the Australian philosopher Julian Savulescu define it.

Moral bioenhancement involves using "pharmacological and genetic methods, like genetic selection and engineering" to improve moral motivation.

Persson and Savulescu argue that our need for moral enhancement is especially dire today. So many of our evolved moral responses worked for eras when we were occasionally throwing spears at each other. But they won't suffice for the moral challenges of the future. To take one of Persson and Savulescu's examples, they seem to leave us short of a moral response to climate change. Effective responses to the climate crisis require levels of cooperation beyond both what we are accustomed to and what is required by common-sense morality. I found their 2012 book, *Unfit for the Future: The Need for Moral Enhancement*, in the Great Library. They write:

Modern scientific technology provides us with many means that could cause our downfall. If we are to avoid causing catastrophe by misguided employment of these means, we need to be morally motivated to a higher degree.

According to them, we need moral bioenhancement to avoid Ultimate Harm, an event that would make "worthwhile life *forever* impossible on this planet." Importantly for our debate, moral enhancement should enable us to make wise choices about enhancement technologies.

Winston: So are there other examples of problems that we could better address with improved moral motivations? I understand the need to avoid Ultimate Harm as Persson and Savulescu define it. Any development that realistically threatens to make worthwhile life forever impossible on this planet would certainly seem to warrant our attention. I can also see how our failures to cooperate may be a significant obstacle blocking action on the climate crisis. But what I'm not seeing is how the climate crisis plausibly threatens that outcome.

Sophie: So you don't think that we should worry so much about Ultimate Harm? How do you figure that? Ultimate Harm does sound quite bad!

Winston: Thanks Sophie. The Intergovernmental Panel on Climate Change (IPCC) has described a number of scenarios. The most pessimistic of these, in which we do very little to arrest the increase of greenhouse gasses, will bring misery to millions. But I don't see anything as dramatic as Persson and Savulescu's Ultimate Harm on the IPCC's list. Worthwhile life continues for the fortunate few who insulate themselves from climate change's effects.

Olen: Human extinction is surely a logically possible effect of climate change. Even if the IPCC assigns a low probability to it, shouldn't we be concerned about that?

Winston: I wonder if that is a rational allocation of our concern. Yes, human extinction would certainly be a bad outcome. But does noting that extinction is a logically possible consequence of climate change suffice to make me worried about it? I don't agree with that. Extinction of the human species is a logically possible consequence of me tying my shoelaces right now. That doesn't mean I should worry about it enough to leave my shoelaces untied.

Olen: (*seeming frustrated*) But human extinction is about as bad an outcome as possible for our species, surely!

Winston: If we worried about any action that is a logically possible cause of extinction then we would be too busy worrying to do anything!

Olen: OK Professor! What according to you is the right way to allocate our concern? You seem to be suggesting that we should worry a great deal about the potential of climate change to immiserate millions, but we shouldn't worry too much about its potential to send us extinct.

Winston: I like the approach of the American psychologist Elke Weber. She presents our collective response to climate change as drawing on a "finite pool of worry" to divide among all our priorities. Weber argues that "Unlike money or other material resources, which can be saved or borrowed, the amount of attention available to anyone to process the vast amount of information potentially available on innumerable topics is small and very finite." What I take out of this is that we shouldn't worry at all about many merely logically possible causes of Ultimate Harm.

Olen: (*sounding sceptical*) So not only are you telling me that you don't fear extinction, you're saying that people concerned for the human species shouldn't.

Winston: That's not what I'm saying at all! I'm saying that we should be guided by rationality in our fears of extinction. Imagine that we allocated worry from what Weber refers to as our finite pool of worry to every logically possible cause of extinction that we believe to be compatible with the laws of physics. We are limited beings with finite resources of worry to distribute. Perhaps the near limitless intellects that you would like exponential tech progress to turn us into, Olen, could worry that someone's tying their shoelaces could cause Ultimate Harm. But merely noting that it's a logically possible cause of extinction shouldn't suffice for us to worry about it. I'm not going to be worried about tying my shoelaces even if you tell me that, for all we know, a shoelace-tying trigger of human extinction *might* be compatible with the laws of physics. There's simply too much for us finite beings to think about today.

Sophie: I'm just trying to get my head around this. Weber's claim about the finitude of our collective worry reminds me a bit about the concern about the drain on children's attention spans due to addictive social media technologies like TikTok. I guess one way to express that concern is to say that children have only a finite amount of attention to direct at learning, family, and friendships. TikTok takes so much of a child's finite pool of attention that it leaves so little for other more important concerns.

Winston: Yes Sophie, that could be a useful analogy.

Olen: So what does this mean for Persson and Savulescu's suggestions about moral bioenhancement as a way to avoid Ultimate Harm?

Winston: Perhaps it's just a framing issue. We should be worried about climate change as a cause of human misery even if we ignore it as cause of Ultimate Harm which, if you remember, makes worthwhile life *forever* impossible on this planet.

Olen: Thank you Winston, I guess. So we might still need moral bioenhancement then? The good news is that we can take our first steps towards a morally bioenhanced future quite soon. There are pharmaceuticals that can equip us to make morally wise choices about increasingly powerful enhancement technologies. Studies suggest that SSRIs widely prescribed for depression may bring additional moral benefits. Some studies suggest that people on SSRIs are more likely to engage in cooperative behaviour than those who aren't.

Winston: So Kramer's cosmetic pharmacology wins after all?

Olen: Remember that Persson and Savulescu aren't arguing for mass prescription of Prozac. They are arguing for a serious research programme that would take the positive effects of SSRIs on moral behaviour as evidence that moral bioenhancers can be developed if we want to and are prepared to invest the money.

Winston: So are there any further suggestions about moral bioenhancers we might develop? I do wonder about philosophers asking for money. Are there signs that biotechnology forms are taking this suggestion seriously? Or is this just a case of academic philosophers asking for money to fly to exotic destinations to give papers at conferences?

Olen: That's unfair Winston. We need philosophers to establish the viability of a project like moral bioenhancement before we commit serious money to it. And I don't see why philosophers shouldn't be allowed to combine work and pleasure by discussing this in Tuscany. But SSRIs aren't the only promising lead. There's also research on oxytocin – the "love drug" or "cuddle hormone." This seems to make us feel closer to each other. Release of oxytocin helps a mother to bond with a newborn. Snorting it in experimental settings seems to help humans to bond with others.

Winston: I think you might be too credulous about what to count as a promising lead. The idea that we can fix moral problems simply by asking Big Pharma to design a fix for us is surely a terrible oversimplification. The Swiss philosopher Fabrice Jotterand points to the complexities in the formation of our moral identities, the influences that make us, morally speaking. He wants the philosophers who argue for these quick fixes to do much more reading in psychiatry.

Olen: Thanks Winston. But I trust the philosophers who argue for moral bioenhancement to keep up to date with the literature on all of the effects of drugs like SSRIs. These philosophers do enlist the support of experts outside of philosophy.

Winston: I am worried about how philosophers read that literature and solicit advice from scientists. When philosophers appoint themselves as advocates of moral bioenhancement there's concern about bias. They will

	tend to mention research that supports their view and omit research that doesn't. But perhaps that's a different issue from the one we are concerned about here.
Olen:	So Jotterand is prepared to accept that moral bioenhancement might be possible. We just have to make sure we prepare for it by relying more on the psychiatrists than on the Big Pharma reps? Perhaps I can accept that. But remember that we are somewhat under the gun here. Exponential progress is bringing powerful enhancement technologies soon!
Winston:	A future in which we are all going to be drugged to improve our moral behaviour? I think I'm going to need antidepressants to live in that world even if they don't morally improve me.
Olen:	Don't worry, Winston. No one will require you to take Prozac to morally improve yourself. You should look at these studies more as a proof of concept. Drugs that are safe enough to be taken by millions of people to treat mood disorders seemingly have effects on moral behaviour. We should look to a future in which we develop drugs that safely boost Prozac's moral effects while reducing unwanted side effects. Might an aerosolized dose of oxytocin strategically sprayed by the United Nations reduce the chances that two nations will go to war with each other?
Eugenie:	I don't want to rain on your parade too much, Olen. But here's something that concerns me about your morally bioenhanced path to global peace. I read that oxytocin is responsive to the distinction between in-group and out-group members. This seems to make sense given what we understand about its biological function. Oxytocin prompts mothers to bond with their own babies. But it doesn't lead to generalized baby-hugging in a maternity ward. Olen, your plan to aerosolize it and apply it to inflamed international border disputes may lead to increased empathy with your fellow soldiers but reduced

empathy for those across the border you're being asked to bomb. I would respectfully suggest that this is not a moral enhancement the world needs right now.

Olen: I am a bit disappointed about how you have responded to my offers of an enhanced future for the human species. I see that Winston has volunteered to choose our next setting. I can't say that I'm looking forward to that!

Night 7　How do we decide which aspects of human nature to preserve?

Coffee in the Bwindi Impenetrable National Park in Uganda

Olen:　　Quite a different setting from the New London of 632 AF! Well I guess the lesson we should learn from this is that tech people can furnish the tools but they don't necessarily get to say how these tools are used – or abused. Winston, why do I think that you were the one who chose this particular coffee venue. I'm wondering what anti-tech diatribe you have in mind?

Winston:　I did choose this locale. But don't worry I'm not going to restrict you to the range of coffees available in the actual Bwindi Impenetrable National Park. We retain access to the Great Library and to the full range of virtual coffees. But yes, I am going to get creative with Olen's digital tech so we can explore some gaps in his human enhancement *über alles* approach.

Olen:　　I'm all ears.

Winston:　A few nights ago you defined radical enhancement as improvement of human capacities to levels far beyond the biologically normal range for human beings. Do you stand by that?

Olen:　　Sure!

DOI: 10.4324/9781003321613-7

The meaning of the luddites

Winston: I've arranged for some mountain gorillas – *Gorilla beringei beringei* – to approach our viewing platform. I want to emphasize that I'm not some luddite opponent of technological progress. I love this aspect of digital tech – lifelike mountain gorillas that peaceably sidle up to us as we are enjoying our very pleasant virtual special coffees, guaranteed to never give us hangovers. My problem is when you think you can direct those same fast-advancing technologies at our biological brains and bodies.

Sophie: OK Winston. I don't think you're a luddite. So what are we supposed to learn from these magnificent virtual specimens? We may have been too reckless with nature to save actual *Gorilla beringei beringei* from extinction, but these magnificent specimens are guaranteed eternal life so long as no one presses the off switch on the Metaverse?

Winston: No, that's not why I brought you here.

Olen: Is this going to be you guilt-tripping us about our desecration of the gorillas' habitat? People like you are far too busy making us feel bad. By the way, I *do* think you're a luddite. In the late 1790s Ned Ludd supposedly smashed two mechanical knitting machines as an act of protest against the Industrial Revolution. We know both that his revolt against progress failed and that it's excellent that it did. Think about the wonderful technologies that Ludd sought to deny us. How many future wonder techs will you cheat us of, Winston?

Winston: I'm definitely not a luddite! My concern is about the powerful digital technologies that you want to direct at our human natures. I want to selectively smash some of those. But I am disappointed about the crude philosophical uses people make of the luddites. Because we think we know how things turned out, we view anyone in history who advanced a contrary view as obviously misguided.

Olen: So how should we be thinking about the luddites, then?

Winston: It would help if we didn't just view them as history's losers. I like the view expressed by the English social historian E. P. Thompson in his 1963 book *The Making of the English Working Class*. He presented the luddites not as fools trying to call a halt to technological progress, but mainly calling for a better deal from it for workers. Perhaps Ned Ludd and his followers are best compared with today's Amazon Fulfilment Centre employees calling for improvements in their pay and work conditions. They really don't want to abolish Amazon.

Olen: (*getting annoyed*) Thanks for the boring history lecture.

Winston: No problem. I'm also disappointed that you think that's the philosophical use I'm going to make of these magnificent virtual beasts.

Should we fix gorillas' problems by uplifting them?

Sophie: So why are you showing them to us, Winston?

Winston: I want you to think about gorillas as candidates for radical cognitive enhancement. One of the selling points of radical cognitive enhancement is supposed to be creating beings who stand to us intellectually as we stand to our apelike ancestors. But I want to turn that point on its head. Perhaps we could radically enhance the intellects of gorillas. We should be asking whether that would really improve their lives.

Eugenie: Winston, what you are discussing is the project of uplifting. Humans aren't the only candidates for enhancement. If humans can benefit from becoming smarter then surely mountain gorillas can too. It's clear that gorillas are victims of shrinking habitats. Humans have been turning remaining gorilla habitats into farmland. I agree that this is a problem and that we should do something about it. Perhaps if we became more solution focused rather than seeking to blame impoverished people for turning gorilla habitat into farmland, then might see a solution for the extinction threat confronting the gorillas in enhancement technologies. Suppose we uplift gorillas. Maybe cognitively enhanced gorillas could join humans in farming the land that we are struggling to preserve as their natural habitats. Humans farm to increase the nutritional yield of land. Gorillas with human-level intelligence could farm too and be that much farther from extinction.

Olen: Welcome back to team enhancement, Eugenie!

Winston: So if I understand the proposal of team enhancement, we should address the challenge faced by mountain gorillas by applying enhancement technologies to them. I'm guessing you are about tell us about humanizing the *Gorilla beringei beringei* genome by editing in genes associated with human intelligence. You'll be asking how many copies of NR2B we can add to the gorilla genome. But if Olen's got anything to do with the conversation, you'll soon be talking about grafting digital technologies to gorilla brains.

Eugenie: (*uncertain what to make of this apparent change of heart*) Umm, welcome to team enhancement, I guess …?

Winston: Sorry to say that this is not why I brought you here. I'd like you to really focus on what's good for the gorillas themselves. Suppose that humanizing gorillas is the only way to save them from extinction. Perhaps that might be the best option for them in the changed global environment of the Anthropocene. But we should also pay attention to what the gorillas will lose from enhancement.

Sophie: Well, if we suppose that gorillas really are doomed in the Anthropocene then enhancement might be the best option for them. Perhaps this is a *reductio ad absurdum* of our current policies on the environment. If the only way to save gorillas is to enhance them then there must be something wrong with the reasoning that brings us to this point.

What would we do to avoid extinction?

Winston: There are many things that humans would do to avoid extinction. The Serbian philosopher Vojin Rakić has described a survival-at-any-cost bias that he proposes skews our responses to future threats. Rakić grounds it in our biology. He suggests that humans as a biological species will do anything to survive. I wonder if this bias has a detrimental effect here. When presented with even the merest possibility of Ultimate Harm we reach for *anything* that might prevent this.

Sophie: I think we need an example here.

Winston: Suppose we realized we had to live underground to avoid extinction from climate change. We might be prepared to do that if it was the only way we could survive. Moreover, we might confidently predict that we would eventually adapt to life underground. Perhaps our distant descendants will become like the Morlocks of H. G. Wells's 1895 novel, *The Time Machine*. Wells imagines a distant future in which humanity has split into two species, one of which, the Morlocks, lives underground emerging only briefly to feed on members of the other species, the Eloi. So long as the Morlocks get enough Eloi to eat, they seem pretty content. Perhaps we could adapt to living underground in the way that Wells imagines the Morlocks doing. We wouldn't have to dine on other human species. But, even so, surely there are things we should regret about losing our former above-ground existences. I think the same warnings apply to gorilla candidates for uplifting.

Olen: OK Winston, tell us precisely what mountain gorillas would be missing out on if they became smart like us. If we were to ask them after the enhancement procedures wouldn't they be grateful? Not only would they be solving the problems of farming, but they'd also be solving the problems of Rubik's cubes.

Winston: (*smirking*) Fortunately gorillas already have opposable thumbs!

Olen: Enough with the flippant comments, Winston. Can you go into a bit of detail about what these gorillas lose simply by becoming smarter? One of the main reasons we send our kids to school is to make them smarter. Are you going to argue that parents might be right to reject education for their children because we deny them the pleasures of being dumber? As gorillas get smarter they will gain the capacity to do a whole lot of new things, many of which they will enjoy. Just becoming smarter won't deprive them of any activities that they were formerly able to do. Suppose we uplifted gorillas giving them the cognitive capacities of human farmers. We wouldn't deprive them of the ability to climb trees. In breaks from tending their crops they can climb as many trees as they like.

Winston: Thanks Olen. But let's think seriously about what these gorillas might lose by becoming as smart as us. For a start, they have relationships with other gorillas that are of great value to them. Some of these relationships are contingent on *not* being as smart as us. Look at Nigel over there. He seems to be enjoying picking bugs out of his mate Suzi's pelt.

Olen: But I don't see how merely being smarter prevents Nigel from dining on Suzi's bugs and still loving it. And suppose the uplifted Nigel no longer wanted to. Couldn't the pleasures of solving Rubik's cubes more than compensate for that loss. Perhaps Nigel will read and understand the Jane Austen novels that Sophie has always been nagging me about. Perhaps he could even read and understand Ray Kurzweil's monumental work *The Singularity is Near*.

Winston: But if you were to ask Nigel about a change that *might* deprive him of this, offering in its place some future pleasure that he's not currently capable of understanding, I'm betting he would express a preference for being unenhanced and continuing to dine on Suzi's bugs. I agree that no one would be stopping an uplifted gorilla from occasionally participating in the pleasures of unenhanced gorillas. But we are imagining a future in which they lose the desire to perform the activity that currently gives them great pleasure. In exchange they might get desires to do things that they can't currently understand. That doesn't sound like an appealing deal to me.

Olen: So you want Nigel to remain dumb simply because in his current cognitively unenhanced state he can't express a preference for all of the pleasures that enhancement would bring?

Winston: Perhaps. But I'm more concerned about what humans can learn from Nigel's case.

Should we want the things we believe our radically enhanced future selves might want?

Sophie: OK Winston, so the challenge is to use the examples of Nigel and Suzi to formulate a philosophical thought experiment to get a better fix on what we humans could gain, and lose, from overuse of all of the enhancement technologies Olen is marketing.

Olen: That's where I'm not following. It may be that Nigel lacks understanding sufficient to consent to the attachment of neuroprostheses to his brain. But we are in a very different position. We are having an informed discussion about a wide range of enhancement technologies. Do you think that human enhancement sceptics understand the techs I and Eugenie have been advocating?

Sophie: I think I understand the broad outlines of your enhancement plan.

Olen: (*looking at his friends and sounding frustrated*) Clearly gorillas lack the understanding to consent to the application of enhancement technologies to them. But have I not made it clear that I want as much enhancement as tech can offer me?

Sophie: I think I follow that. If you are determined to be one of the risk pioneers that Buchanan celebrates, then good for you. Elon Musk wants to settle human colonists on Mars. I am supposing that the first generations of settlers will be risk pioneers who understand that they may end up dead soon after arrival on the red planet. Might it be the same with enhancement technologies? Would you accept that philosophical compromise, Olen?

Olen: The philosophical shit stirrer in me is annoyed by your insouciant acquiescence to that. I want to follow the reasoning of Bostrom and go further. I want to accept the offer of radical enhancement not just for me, but for you sceptics too. Bostrom enlists the dispositional theory of value proposed by the philosopher David Lewis. He thinks that our values are posthuman even if we aren't yet.

Sophie: (*looks perplexed*) So even Winston wants to become a posthuman? He's an aspiring posthuman in denial? How do you figure that?

Olen: Bostrom thinks that if you really understood what it was that you were forgoing you would want it too. According to the dispositional theory "something is a value for you if and only if you would want it if you were perfectly acquainted with it and you were thinking and deliberating as clearly as possible about it." Suppose your drunken friend expresses a desire to drive home. You can justify appropriating her keys on the grounds that her more rational, sober self would not want to drive home in this state. That rational self would presumably not want to get arrested – or to risk killing someone.

Sophie: So how does the dispositional theory show that Winston really wants to be radically enhanced even if he denies it, or represses this desire?

Olen: Well, just as your drunk friend should comply with the desires of her sober self, Winston's unenhanced self should defer to the desires of his radically enhanced future self. Winston's clearly a smart guy, but his radically enhanced future self knows more than him. The German philosopher Stefan Lorenz Sorgner thinks that we signed up to integrate tech into our natures a long time ago. Enhancement technologies may seem radically new but they are really business as usual for our species.

Winston: Since I seem to be the subject of this discussion let me say that I'm very suspicious about this reasoning.

Olen: Perhaps I should put this another way. Suppose we were to radically enhance Nigel. He then loses interest in dining on Suzi's bugs. Instead he enjoys reading Proust. Would he choose to revert to his unenhanced gorilla state having sampled the joys offered by his cognitively enhanced state? I strongly suspect he would be as willingly to surrender his knowledge of *À la Recherche du Temps Perdu* as Sophie would be to choose to suffer brain damage that would render her insensible to the joys of reading *Pride and Prejudice*.

Sophie: (*looks aghast*) That is a truly horrible thought, Olen. Thanks for including me as a character in your philosophical speculations. Winston, you seem to have directed your avatar to adopt the pose of Auguste Rodin's sculpture *The Thinker*.

Winston: (*unfolding from his* The Thinker *pose*) Thank you Sophie. I think there are things that we would lose from great degrees of enhancement that these breezy stories and counterfactuals tend to overlook. Some losses occur in respect of relationships. Look at Nigel and Suzi. They seem to care about each other. We've been talking about Nigel's pleasure from dining on Suzi's bugs. But really his entire relationship with Suzi is at stake. I think that the losses will be greater for human subjects of enhancement than they would be for Nigel.

Olen: What if Suzi also signed up for cognitive enhancement and became a fan of Austen? You and I are friends Sophie! Surely valued relationships could survive. I'm imagining Nigel and Suzi joining a book club and getting into intense debates about what to make of the 2009 Austen parody novel, *Pride and Prejudice and Zombies*.

Winston: (*sounding exasperated*) Note that you say Nigel and Suzi's relationship "*could* survive." It's too tempting and easy for philosophers to invent stories in which an unprecedented event takes place and everything turns out peachy! But this is an egregious abuse of the philosophical method when applied to the future. The same attitude that directs us to keep emitting carbon and even accelerate our emissions because there *could* be a 2030s climate tech that safely extracts atmospheric carbon restoring Earth to the climate of the 1700s encourages recklessness in respect of enhancement technologies. They *could* produce gloriously happy superintelligent posthumans. We can certainly tell logically coherent stories in which somewhat happy humans are all seamlessly replaced by extremely happy posthumans.

Sophie: So what should we as human candidates for radical enhancement take out of the story about gorilla uplifting? I think I speak for Olen here when I say that I'm not yet convinced that we couldn't continue to enjoy our current pleasures even as radical cognitive enhancement gives us the capacity to play ten-dimensional chess.

Winston: No disrespect to Nigel and Suzi, but human relationships are so much emotionally and cognitively richer than theirs. I've belaboured the point about Nigel's affection for Suzi centring on his enjoyment of her bugs.

But human relationships involve so much more than happy gorilla relationships. Human lovers do occasionally groom each other. But they also go on hikes, join book clubs, play contract bridge, form violin quartets, and debate the philosophy of Friedrich Nietzsche.

Sophie: So is the point that humans have so much more to lose from the overuse of enhancement technologies?

Winston: (*forms* The Thinker *pose again*) I do think that the risks for humans from radical enhancement are greater than for gorillas. The greater richness of our relationships means that we have much more to lose from big uncontrolled changes of the kind a risk pioneer might make. Shouldn't we demand more than the logical possibility that a valued relationship survives a significant change – supposing that we actually care about it? Too many philosophical thought experiments trade on the mere logical possibility that some valued aspects of human existence can survive a big change. You all know that my husband Robert is also an academic. Imagine Robert and I were offered better jobs at more prestigious universities. If we really cared about each other, which I assure you we do, then before we accepted job offers we should at least take an interest in where they are geographically. We would be interested in solving what academic couples refer to as the "two body problem" – finding positions that are in the same place. We surely wouldn't just accept the new offers by reply email and be content about the logical possibility that they will be at universities that are within an easy commute from each other.

Olen: Fair enough, Winston. You've made it clear that you love Robert. What would you say about my attitude to enhancement and my relationship? You know that I just got married to Rachel. We are very much in love. I used my newly minted fortune to sign Rachel up for the Life Extension Foundation, Alcor. It offers cryonics.

Should she suffer some significant mishap and be pronounced dead, Alcor will retrieve her body and preserve it in liquid nitrogen. She and I will await restoration at a time when medicine has advanced to the point of fixing whatever legally killed us. Rachel shares my enthusiasm about radical cognitive enhancement too.

Winston: I'm very happy for you and Rachel. Robert and I sent a card. But given what I've just said about radical cognitive enhancement, I wonder which love is greater. Your love for Rachel or your love of enhancement. I'm not sure if I remembered to add that to my card. I suppose that if you and Rachel share that attitude toward each other and to enhancement then that's fine.

Olen: Well, I share the attitude of my former enhancement ally Eugenie toward personal choice. I guess I can no sooner force you and Robert to enhance yourselves than I can require you to sign up for Alcor. But I do think you're missing out.

Winston: Olen, you say that Robert and I are missing out on the joys of a potentially wonderful future. I accuse you and Rachel of being shallow in your feelings for each other. Perhaps we will have to leave it at that.

Do philosophers' thought experiments about the future encourage recklessness?

Sophie: Winston, you've been talking about enhancement technologies in ways that differ from Olen and the transhumanist advocates of radical enhancement. You've been talking about risk and reckless attitudes toward it.

Winston: Thank you Sophie. Philosophers tend to apply the test of logical possibility to stories about the future and this sets them, and the rest of us, up for disaster. Philosophical thought experiments are a fun game and they serve many legitimate purposes in philosophy but they encourage recklessness when applied to the future.

I suspect that philosophers are far too easily co-opted by commercial interests marketing tech at us.

Olen: (*scowling*) Sounds a bit like the makings of a mad conspiracy theory to me!

Winston: When philosophers are told they can tell any imaginable story about the future and call it a philosophical thought experiment so long as it is logically coherent they are encouraged to speculate in reckless ways.

Olen: This sounds mad to me. But please continue. Can you give me an example of how philosophers' probing of the future with thought experiments encourages recklessness?

Winston: Sure Olen, how about this thought experiment. It's not directly related to human enhancement, but it does show what can go wrong when we place too much faith in stories about the future. (*Winston gestures and text appears.*)

Olen's Tesla: Imagine you are contentedly driving your beautiful Tesla along a road and come across a bridge that looks infirm. You wonder whether you should risk your life and more importantly your technological marvel of a car on the bridge. One thing you might do is get out of your car and inspect the bridge. If you are in doubt and have an engineer friend you might ask them. But that takes time, and you are in a hurry, so instead you avail yourself of the philosopher's method of testing future scenarios by formulating thought experiments. You pause for a couple of minutes before you cross. You imagine how the imminent future might turn out. You're keen to cross the bridge so you conjure up a thought experiment in which your Tesla crosses the bridge without mishap. You do your due diligence as a philosopher and probe your thought experiment for any logical inconsistencies or violations of laws of nature. You find none. So you cross the bridge, which promptly collapses. You die, but fortunately your Tesla is easily salvaged.

Olen:　Obviously that's a foolish way to think about whether it's safe to cross a bridge. But I don't see how it applies to radical human enhancement.

Winston:　I'm sorry to say that it does. Many of our most talented philosophers of enhancement take the same approach to humanity's enhanced future as the Tesla driver does in that thought experiment. If you are in doubt here's a passage from the Oxford philosopher Bostrom. Unsurprisingly, he's one of your heroes Olen. I call him radical enhancement's fabulist-in-chief. Here's Bostrom's story about our radically enhanced future. It almost makes a believer of me. But then I think – I don't want to be like that Tesla driver. Here Bostrom invites his readers to imagine the thrills of radical enhancement.

You have just celebrated your 170th birthday and you feel stronger than ever. Each day is a joy. You have invented entirely new art forms, which exploit the new kinds of cognitive capacities and sensibilities you have developed. You still listen to music – music that is to Mozart what Mozart is to bad Muzak. You are communicating with your contemporaries using a language that has grown out of English over the past century and that has a vocabulary and expressive power that enables you to share and discuss thoughts and feelings that unaugmented humans could not even think or experience. You play a certain new kind of game which combines VR-mediated artistic expression, dance, humor, interpersonal dynamics, and various novel faculties and the emergent phenomena they make possible, and which is more fun than anything you ever did during the first hundred years of your existence. When you are playing this game with your friends, you feel how every fiber of your body and mind is stretched to its limit in the most creative and imaginative way, and you are creating new realms of abstract and concrete beauty that humans could never (concretely) dream of. You are always ready to feel with those who suffer misfortunes, and to work hard to help them get back on their feet. You are also involved in a large voluntary organization that works to reduce suffering of animals in their natural environment in ways that permit ecologies to continue to function in traditional ways; this involves political efforts combined with advanced science and information processing services. Things are getting better, but already each day is fantastic.

Winston: It goes on.

Olen: That's fine, Winston, but I don't see what's wrong with adopting an optimistic mindset toward the future. We've just come through a hideous pandemic. Why can't we join Bostrom in hoping for a wonderfully enhanced future?

Winston: We can certainly hope. But we must be aware that we are *just* hoping. And sometimes just hoping sets us up for disappointment and disaster. I think that an attitude of overconfidence in our technologies and technological progress in general is part of the explanation why some of the most technologically advanced nations suffered the highest pandemic death tolls. We underestimated SARS-Cov-2 *and* we overestimated the powers of our techs. Overreliance on the stories of would-be radical enhancers like Bostrom mean that we set ourselves up for disappointment about the technologies we apply to ourselves. It's one thing to be wrong about a virus, quite another to be wrong about potentially irreversible changes to the fundaments of our human natures.

From surveillance capitalism to enhancement capitalism?

Sophie: The political scientist Philip Tetlock warns us about the dangers of overconfident predictions of future events. I wonder if there is a different kind of philosophical overconfidence that a twenty-first century Socrates might warn us about.

Winston: We've had far too many transhumanist thought experiments. I think you know my views about them. They

Olen:

are little more than crude marketing. Here's a bioconservative thought experiment that will illuminate things overlooked by transhumanists' marketing spiels.

Olen:
Let's hear your anti-marketing thought experiment Winston. I'm going to prepare myself by dialling up some powerful antidepressant effects on my neural lace.

Winston: I'm sad to hear that you find the human condition so depressing.

Olen:
Being human is fine, but there really is something so, so much better.

Winston: Here's my anti-marketing enhancement thought experiment.

Beware the wisdom of future philosophers: Suppose there is a neuroprosthesis that once inserted significantly enhances its recipient's ability to perform mental calculations. For example, recipients of the chip can render the cubed root of 1,213,955,826,768,261 within a microsecond. Those who have this neuroprosthesis inserted enjoy significant economic advantages. They do better at school. They get higher paying jobs. Once these labour market advantages become apparent the new enhancement technology is inserted by those who can afford it. The neuroprosthesis has other effects. Studies confirm that recipients of the neuroprosthesis are much less likely to indulge in aimless imaginative reveries than members of the control group without the chip. When pressed to attempt these directionless acts of imagination the recipients of the neuroprosthesis find that they really can't. The inventors of the neuroprosthesis consider this capacity to be worth sacrificing to gain the obvious economic benefits of the neuroprosthesis. But the experimenters don't act in the reckless way as He Jiankui did in his ethically unsupervised gene-editing experiment. They seek approval from the ethical experts. The bioethicists address the loss of the capacity for aimless reverie and consider whether it is worth sacrificing to achieve the obvious benefits brought by the new enhancement tech. These philosophical experts consult all the dominant ethical theories extant at the commencement of the Age of Human Enhancement. They offer their professional verdict that what is gained is worth much more than what is lost and so grant approval.

Olen: Sounds good to me. I like the way you've introduced the bioethicists. They are normally the people that tech types like me are accused of ignoring. Who could complain about that?

Winston: I will clarify the thought experiment's philosophical implications. When we apply radical enhancement technologies to our natures we, in effect, place a bet on what matters about being human. The imagined chip radically enhances subjects' capacity to do long division. This is an obvious improvement. We lose the ability to perform some trivial mental act. We consult our best theories about what matters about being human and confirm that this loss doesn't matter much. I'm concerned about the momentous nature of the experiment and the approval granted by the bioethicists.

Olen: So why are you so sure the chip would spread across the entire population? Isn't it more likely that some people will try it for them and their kids? Others will refrain.

Winston: It's important to not overlook the economic pressures on individuals making these choices in the Age of Human Enhancement. I speculate that the chip will be expensive to begin with, but once the economic advantages become apparent it will swiftly be adopted by almost everyone who has access to it. But this is not a prediction.

Olen: Not a prediction? So just a story?

Winston: It is just a story, but the kind of story we will need to hear as the Age of Human Enhancement gets underway. There's a difference between a prediction about the Age of Human Enhancement and a speculation about how things could go in it. We need many conjectures as we enter an intrinsically uncertain future. They serve as a form of philosophical insurance against things turning out much worse than any of our appointed experts predict. Suppose that kids with the new chip easily outperform their unenhanced classmates and easily get into prestigious professional programmes at universities. Suppose also that few of them bother to study philosophy. I think there's a good chance that liberal democratic states will be pressured into subsidizing the chip for those who cannot afford it. Of course, acceptance may not be universal, at least to begin with. There will be some who reject the chip for themselves and for their children. But they are likely to be increasingly marginalized.

Olen: I prefer my optimistic stories to your depressing ones.

Winston: Your optimistic stories will be excellent ways to sell future enhancement technologies. I think you'll do well pitching them to companies that will emerge to sell us this tech. Shoshanna Zuboff writes about a surveillance capitalism in which companies like Facebook/Meta and Google enjoy unprecedented access to our purchasing intentions. They supplement this with a capacity to profitably influence our behaviour. A superficial understanding of what it means to be human will see us binning aspects of our humanity that, if we thought seriously about them, we would preserve. We should be concerned that Zuboff's surveillance capitalism will be followed by an even more unsettling enhancement capitalism. If surveillance capitalism makes billionaires, enhancement capitalism could make trillionaires. But that could be good news for you and your optimistic stories, Olen. If my speculation comes to pass there will be lots to money to pay you to tell your feel-good stories about enhancement tech. They'll make great marketing copy!

Olen: But you're not certain about any of this?

Winston: Olen, your stories about the future manifest a great deal of confidence about the development of technologies that we might apply to our human natures. I'm suggesting we need to put equal effort into imagining the decisions that humans will make when offered these diverse enhancement technologies. Olen, you appeal to Moore's Law to make your technological forecasts. My story draws on the momentous nature of introducing new enhancement techs. It calls for imaginative engagement with the decisions we might make. Some of these could make irreversible changes to what it means to be human.

Philosophical uncertainty about what it means to be human

Olen: But the relevant experts, the professional ethicists, have green-lit the procedure. What more could you ask?

Winston: My thought experiment draws on philosophical uncertainty about what matters about being human. The questions of what it means to be human and what matters about being human are philosophical perennials. The philosophers of ancient Greece gave different answers from the philosophers of the Enlightenment. Fortunately, these views about what matters about being human are well represented in the academy that produces most of today's ethical experts. There are theorists who defend virtue ethical views derived from the ancient Greeks. There are defenders of the utilitarian and Kantian views of the European Enlightenment. But these draw on a narrow sample of views about what matters about being human. Even within the European tradition the views expressed by the ethical experts who find themselves on committees that grant approval for interventions tend to be secular. We don't hear as much from religious thinkers. But this is only the beginning of a complaint about the biased sample of views about what matters about being human.

Eugenie: Uh-oh, Winston's on a roll!

Winston: I thought it was important to acknowledge and address my own Eurocentric bias. I have to confess ignorance about the assessments of Māori Tohunga, the sages of Kenya, the Sensei of Japan, and the Xiansheng of China about what it is to be human and what matters about it. This momentous change for the entire human species will be occurring with insufficient ethical input from them.

Olen: Well done, Winston. You've just established your politically correct credentials and are guaranteed to be granted tenure at your university!

Winston: Well done back, Olen. Especially on the expression of contempt you've arranged for your avatar to express. I'm just pointing to a risk. Today's ethics committees may find little value in the aimless reverie that our hypothetical neuroprosthesis eliminates. But we are currently sampling a narrow range of ethical opinion. I heartily endorse the willingness to listen to other views about what matters that I'm supposing your moan about political correctness is meant to dismiss. I may know little about the ethical views of Māori Tohunga. But I and they are human. So when they present ethical views my human brain is built to understand them. When I hear them I can be persuaded by them. But I have to hear them first. How do I know that deep within a Chinese ethical tradition is a view by a Xiansheng about aimless reverie that, that if I got to hear it would persuade me that even the great economic advantages brought by the chip don't justify deleting this seemingly pointless capacity. Remember that we are supposing that the economic advantages of the chip are significant enough for it to promptly spread throughout the entirety of humanity.

Sophie: There is a lot of literature to scroll through here. I was grateful that the memory enhancement that came with the neural lace enabled me to cope with the extensive literature in the Western tradition. I have come across some interesting contributions on the ethics of gene editing from Māori scholars. Maui Hudson has written about the relevance of Māori thinking to questions about whether we should use gene editing as an enhancement technology. He points to the importance of *whakapapa,* which translates into English as ancestry or genealogy, to the use of gene editing as an enhancement technology. The modification of your genetic material has the potential to weaken important connections with ancestors and with other people today connected to you by that ancestry.

Olen: So if I'm not Māori how is this relevant to me?

Sophie: Well you are human aren't you? You should at least consider these values before you embark on a path of human enhancement that may weaken your and your descendants' abilities to understand them. But I should confess that this broadening of the scope of ethical consideration has overwhelmed me somewhat. I do agree with Winston that the excuse that we didn't read it because we were just too busy thinking about other issues, issues that seemed more important at the time, isn't great. We will stand indicted by the moral judges of future ages if we overlook issues that they find very important just because we couldn't be bothered to think about them. Perhaps the moral judges of 2050 will have more time to consider the appraisals of enhancement technologies that professional ethicists at the outset of the Age of Human Enhancement dismissed as unimportant.

Eugenie: Perhaps we need a global survey of opinions about what matters about being human.

Olen: Easily done! I'll design a Facebook survey. Facebook may currently be losing users to other social media platforms but it still has a big enough share of the global population to attempt such a survey. Once the data are gathered and processed we can happily turn human enhancement into an engineering problem.

Winston: What we need must go considerably beyond a social media survey. I can imagine how Facebook might run such a survey – "The following is a list of attributes that some people say they value about being human. Rank their importance to you from 1 to 100." This would almost certainly generate a great deal of data quite efficiently. But it falls far short of what we need. People must reflect deeply on what they value about being human and which parts they'd give up if the inducements from enhancement tech are sufficient.

Eugenie: So we need to think more deeply about what we value about the human condition. Do you think this is likely to happen?

Winston: There are twin challenges for any such attempt to understand our values before we enhance them out of existence.

Sophie: What are these twin challenges, Winston?

Winston: First, current trends in university funding and priorities aren't helping. One of the traditional focuses of university teaching and research has been the humanities, academic disciplines that study human society and culture. Yet these are areas that are currently being cut so that more money can be spent on STEM subjects – science, technology, engineering, and mathematics. To some politicians these subjects are all about the future. If we don't support the humanities we will lose that capacity to seriously investigate human values. When we turn techs produced by STEM subjects inward at our human natures we'll be clueless about what to preserve.

Sophie: Well in an ideal world we would have many humanities scholars working on which aspects of our humanity most need defence against enhancement tech. But we don't inhabit that ideal world, Winston, so we must do our best.

Winston: Then there's the other challenge. The defunding of the humanities occurs at a time in which tech companies are getting better and better at selling stuff to us. As we gain this knowledge we should understand the skill with which technology companies market their products. I've expressed my concern that the Age of Human Enhancement will see an enhancement capitalism in which corporations get better at selling us enhancement technologies. Perhaps the trillionaires of a 2040 human enhancement economy will look back on the centibillionaires of the 2020s digital economy in the way they in turn look back on the single billion of John D. Rockefeller Snr's oil refining business.

Sophie: Winston, I'm persuaded by your point about tech promises that aren't realized. I've seen many potential cures for diabetes fail to eventuate. So I cultivate what I think is a healthy scepticism about Olen's exponentially improving enhancement technologies.

Sophie: Well, Winston suggested that concerns about the application of enhancement technologies might be available to us if we read more broadly. Perhaps if we invested less of our energy engaging other viewpoints in our Western traditions then we might be able to make time to consider non-Western views about the importance of being human and remaining so. Perhaps the philosophers of the future will be dismayed at the energy Kantians invested in arguing which version of the Categorical Imperative best describes the obligations of prospective parents interested in enhancement combined with the extreme lack of regard for the concerns raised by thinkers outside of that tradition. These non-Westerners thought hard about what it means to be human. And the choices we make today about which enhancement technologies to apply to our human natures concern them. The enhancement technologies that people get in California will soon be arriving in Aotearoa New Zealand.

Olen: This sounds far too politically correct to me!

Sophie: Perhaps the lesson is that we should listen to Socrates and avoid philosophical overconfidence. Suppose the best bioethical theories of 2050 find the capacity for aimless reverie to be among the most valuable of all human mental abilities. Perhaps we couldn't have predicted this. But we can at least say that we were cautious in our dismissal of aimless reverie. Rather than saying "It has no value according to our dominant philosophical views so it can safely be eradicated in the pursuit of enhanced mathematical abilities" we might instead say "We can't yet see much value in the capacity for aimless reverie. But it does seem to be something that humans do quite a lot of. So let's be cautions in how our enhancement technologies might molest it."

Olen: So what are we supposed to learn from this? If we are too utopian about future technologies we might make mistakes that cannot be reversed?

Winston: I think that the lesson should be that we shouldn't get too carried away by the marketing pitches of those who want to fundamentally change our basic natures. When we hear pitches from tech people they are often trying to sell us something. Let's not be too credulous about what they are offering. Especially given that we may have an incomplete picture of what it is that we are being asked to renounce.

Olen: (*looks bored*) Winston, we've basically stopped listening to you. Can I just observe that your go-slow approach to technological progress and enhancement technologies won't win in the end? I predict that recognition of the chip's economic advantages means that many will adopt it. So you'll just need to get used to it.

Winston: Perhaps you're right if we're making forecasts about the adoption of new enhancement technologies. But that doesn't make human enhancement the morally or prudentially right thing to do. Thrasymachus, one of the characters in Plato's *Republic*, defends the view that "might makes right." Socrates rightly rebuts that. You're effectively saying that economic advantage makes right. I think this is mistaken for similar reasons. We may predict that the mighty and the economically advantaged typically win disputes but that doesn't make them right.

Sophie: That's enough for now. Our focus has been on the big picture of radical enhancement. I think we need to narrow our focus to consider the implications of radical enhancement for individuals.

Winston: Sorry Olen, but I have more to say. Radical enhancement is a transformative change.

Olen: Sounds like you're ready to explore the wonderful potential of the Singularity for human nature!

Winston: Not quite. I'm going to choose tomorrow night's venue to explore a different concern about too much human enhancement.

Night 8   A species relativist rejection of radical enhancement

Coffee outside a cyberconversion facility on the Planet Mondas

Olen: This is ... not what I was expecting. It's a combination of futuristic and shoddily constructed kitsch.

Winston: Welcome to a Metaverse extrapolation of the set of the only TV sci-fi series I ever enjoyed, the BBC's *Dr Who*. You are on planet Mondas as depicted in a 1966 episode of the show – "The Tenth Planet." Mondas is a twin planet of Earth peopled by beings exactly like humans. These Mondasians do as Olen thinks we should and apply a variety of enhancement technologies to their biological natures. A process known as cyberconversion turns Mondasians into Cybermen, the show's second most featured baddies, after the iconic Daleks. Cyberconversion "upgrades" humans by extracting their brains and rehousing them in machine exoskeletons. The process is accompanied by screams giving evidence that the human candidate for cyberconversion remains conscious throughout the procedure. A collection of distinctively human values is replaced by a collection of values oriented toward domination of the galaxy and cyberconverting more humans.

Olen: I hope that your endorsement of *Dr Who*'s attitude toward science doesn't carry over to its philosophical recommendations. I see that the human inhabitants of

DOI: 10.4324/9781003321613-8

this twin Earth somehow survived even after Mondas departed its orbit around the sun, traversing deep space.

Winston: Clearly it's a thought experiment, and a useful one for our purposes.

Is radical enhancement a transformative change?

Olen: We should be careful about what we learn from this fanciful story. Have you just browsed the internet for any fiction that presents the fusion of human and machine in an unflattering light? I think this discussion would go so much better if only I could persuade you to swallow some happy pills.

Winston: Viewers of *Dr Who* see cyberconversion being imposed on humans. But it is made clear that this is not now the process began. The first Cybermen originated from humans who freely chose the path Olen advocates us taking. Their original applications of technology to themselves are born out of the desire to live longer and be smarter. The lesson from the series is they pay an immense price to achieve these ends. They require special technologies known as inhibitors to suppress their human emotions. Otherwise they would presumably flee this chosen technological nightmare. Suicide would be preferable. But, with their emotions suppressed, they continue on their path of galactic domination.

Olen: Well the Cybermen clearly don't fit with my vision of the posthuman future. Affectively enhanced posthumans won't need any of these inhibitors you are imagining to do the right thing. Their natural states will be joyful, upbeat, and productive.

Winston: There's the overconfidence about the future of a tech dude whose company is a unicorn.

Olen: This does come back to your curmudgeonly state Winston. Why all the doom and gloom? Hollywood knows that dystopian sci-fi sells. *Dr Who*'s screenplays are written for human audiences who clearly won't watch a TV series whose message is that there's something better than being human. Since you're trying to turn this serious debate into an argument about which sci-fi character is best, I'm going to register my preference for Data, the charming beneficent cyborg who strolled the bridge of the USS *Enterprise* (NCC-1701-D). I don't see why adding chips and digital prosthetics to our natures couldn't make us more like him. I bet Data wouldn't have any difficulty both understanding that climate change is an existential threat for humanity and acting to prevent and reverse it.

Winston: I'm going to use this setting to explore a different issue. I'm interested in the extent to which we as individuals benefit from changes like cyberconversion. The Mondasians go through something I'll call a *transformative change*. I suggest that radical enhancement is a species of transformative change. This is what makes it philosophically problematic.

Olen: Transformative change – sounds like philosophers' gobbledegook to me.

Winston: Here's a definition that I find helpful: "A transformative change alters the state of an individual's mental or physical characteristics in a way that causes and warrants a significant change in how that individual evaluates a wide range of their own experiences, beliefs, or achievements."

Olen: I'm just trying to work out how this helps with our evaluation of radical enhancement. I just Googled "transformative experiences" and came across the work of the philosopher Laurie Paul. Paul writes illuminatingly about her experiences of being pregnant and becoming a parent for the first time. She labels pregnancy and giving birth as transformative experiences because they can change beliefs about whether it's a good idea to become a parent. Also, you can't really know what these experiences are like until you've had them. You cannot know until you've had them whether becoming a parent is a good idea, but once you've gotten pregnant and given birth it's too late. Here's what Paul says about transformative experiences: (*Olen gestures and text appears.*)

not only do you not know the values before you've had the relevant experience, but having the experience can change your preferences, and so the values you would (*per impossibile*) assign these outcomes before having the transformative experience could be radically different from the values you'd assign to the relevant outcomes after having had the experience. So because you don't know what the experience is like, you don't know how your preferences will change as a result of having the transformative experience.

Eugenie: Could you explain the relevance of that to enhancement?
Olen: Now, Paul certainly doesn't say this. But perhaps radical enhancement is a transformative experience. We can't know what it's like ahead of doing it. But becoming a parent turned out well for her. She took a leap into the dark and the result was good. Perhaps we should take a leap into the dark with radical enhancement and expect that it will turn out well?
Eugenie: That sounds a bit reckless, Olen. Pregnancy turned out well for Paul. But there are transformative experiences that have negative consequences. There are people who regret becoming parents even if it's not common to publicly confess it. It is possible to both love your children and regret becoming a parent. But you can see how expressing that might puzzle your children. "Hi kids, I love you and would do almost anything to ensure your flourishing, but I do regret your very existence. I would have preferred to continue the carefree life I had before you."

Winston: I wonder if this focus on experiences whose quality you can't predict is a bit of a red herring. The Swedish philosopher Krister Bykvist objects to Paul, believing that even if we can't know *for sure* what the experience of being a parent for the first time is like before you've done it, there are sources of information available about it. These fall short of certainty but that's true of many of our claims to know things. Paul could have asked friends of hers what it's like to be a parent before she took the plunge. That doesn't give her the full picture of what it's like, but it's still useful and can support an informed choice.

Eugenie: So how's what you are saying about transformative change different?

Winston: I'm not supposing that you can't know how you will assess radical enhancement until you've undergone it. You can ask people who've applied enhancement technologies to their bodies or psyches and ask them how they feel about it. If they inform you that they are loving being enhanced then perhaps that's something to inform a forecast about how radical enhancement will be for you. Perhaps you should be confident that you will love your new supersmart state. Nevertheless, I think you should muster the confidence to reject it, your confident forecast notwithstanding.

Eugenie: This all sounds a bit mystical to me. You accept that you won't suffer buyer's remorse about radical enhancement. So why not do it?

Winston: Because it goes against my deep values about how I as a human should be.

Eugenie: You're going to have to walk me through an example or two here.

Winston: Sure. If radical enhancement is a transformative change then it may alter subjects' deepest values. This explains why it can be perfectly appropriate for me to reject radical cognitive enhancement even if I understand that were I to mistakenly swallow radical enhancement pills I would be very happy with the results. Perhaps I can offer my relationship with Robert as an example? Do you believe me when I affirm my love for him?

Olen: Of course. But I do think we are hearing too much about your and Robert's amazing relationship.

Winston: What do you think would happen to that relationship if I were to radically enhance my intellect but Robert were to reject enhancement? I predict that Robert's conversational barbs that currently amuse me greatly would from that enhanced perspective just seem trite. I might still like Robert but it's hard to imagine our relationship surviving in anything like its current form.

Olen: Surely if you love each other you'll sign up together. The enhancement facilities of the future will offer well-priced his-and-his packages.

Winston: I follow that. But I'm still not confident it would be good for our relationship. Perhaps I can draw your attention back to the title of Bostrom's article "Why I Want to be a Posthuman When I Grow Up." One thing I remember about all of the friendships I formed at school is that none of them survived into adulthood. We went off and did different things and basically fell out of touch. I wouldn't be at all confident of reforming the friendships of my youth founded on building increasingly elaborate tracks for our toy trains. I think of Robert and me as grown up. Radical cognitive enhancement does offer some benefits, but suppose we were both of go through the degree of enhancement that typically occurs today when children grow up. Radically enhanced Winston and radically enhanced Robert might have about as much interest in each other as I currently have for the people I used to assemble toy train tracks with when we were kids. Sorry but Robert and I are more in love with each other than we are in the human enhancement project.

Olen: Can you give another example not mawkishly focused on your love for Robert?

Could you take a pill that made you a racist?

Winston: Here's another thought experiment that will test your commitment to the idea that we should go with the assessment of our future enhanced selves. You're not going to enjoy it! Suppose I designed a pill that would alter you psychologically so you became a white supremacist. Could I interest you in that?

Olen: (*looking aghast*) That's an horrific prospect!

Winston: Of course, I agree. But imagine I did design this pill and you mistakenly took it. I then ask you whether you are happy you did so. Can you see that future Nazi Olen would answer that question differently from the way you do now? You're very smart, Olen, but I'm sure if we went back in time and submitted some of the leading members of Germany's Nazi Party in the 1930s to psychometric tests we would probably find some impressive IQs. Despite what we might like to think, high intelligence offers no immunity against morally obnoxious views. Once you'd been psychologically Nazified, you might even thank me for an intervention that truly opened your eyes to the ways of the world. You'd enthusiastically seek out the social media platforms with the greatest representation of white supremacist views. When on them you'd write ecstatically about your "awakening." If anyone asked you if you had any regrets you'd say "Definitely not!" and offer the procedure as a fix for any doubts about the supremacy of the white race.

Olen: Winston, this is nightmarish. Not only do I strongly want it to not happen I don't want to be the subject of any more of your sadistic thought experiments.

Winston: I'm not finished yet – time to harvest more philosophical implications of my *Olen Thought Experiment*. Do you mind if I call it that? If I publish this thought experiment in a journal it will need a memorable name.

Olen: Please don't call it that! I'm wondering if my patent lawyer handles defamation cases.

Winston: Of course, the suggestion that I have this neurotech and could apply it to you constitutes no argument in favour of white supremacy. All I'm saying is that undergoing this transformation will predictably change the way you evaluate the change. A transformation that you view as a prudential harm – a change that made you worse off – before you undergo it will be viewed as a transformation that improves your well-being after you have undergone it. You'll seek out new friends who confirm your new ethical views. These friendships will become very meaningful for you in a world that is so hostile to your new beliefs.

Olen: My first question is – how is this relevant to the debate about radical enhancement? My second question is how much money will you accept to never make me the subject of further morally disgusting thought experiments?

Winston: No worries, I can promise that there will be no Olen transformative change thought experiments, published by me at least. Anyway, journals take so long to publish that I will have moved on before any editor agrees to publish this thought experiment. My broader point is that radical enhancement could be a bit like this. Our possible radically enhanced future selves would predictably be very pleased to have undergone this change but that fact constitutes no argument for accepting radical enhancement.

Eugenie: I'm not sure I want to get in the middle of this Winston-Olen fight. But I am thinking that my approach with its emphasis on moderate enhancement, the kind of enhancement that might be achieved by tweaking a single gene that influences the development of the human brain, might be the most prudent approach. It's certainly a way to reduce the possibility of some of the extreme tech derangements of human nature that worry Winston.

A kind of species relativism?

Sophie: Winston, I think we need some philosophical termi- nology to describe the view that you are defending. It sounds a bit like a relativist position. In philosophy we are trained to feel contempt for any kind of rela- tivism. Sometimes a student might say in a Philosophy 101 class – "Well murder might be morally wrong for you, but perhaps it's not morally wrong for others." Sometimes the student will claim to remember a story about a distant culture that morally endorses murder. Would you accept a description of your view as a kind of relativism, Winston?

Winston: Perhaps it is a kind of relativism. I am saying that some value judgments right for radically enhanced posthu- mans aren't right for unenhanced humans. The lesson of our trip to the virtual Bwindi Impenetrable National Park was that some experiences properly valued by gorillas aren't valuable to humans. And vice versa. The kind of species relativism suggests that we shouldn't be convinced by the rapturous assessments of radically enhanced humans about their lives. I also suspect that any time-travelling prehumans shouldn't be too upset by our suggestions that we think it's better to be human than prehuman. Those assessments have nothing to do with the lived experiences of prehumans.

Eugenie: Does this species relativism have similar implications to the kinds of cultural relativism that philosophers have long dismissed?

Winston: I think that's a useful comparison. There's a national rel- ativism in the teams we cheer for in the football World Cup. Nigerians tend to support the Nigerian team and

Finns the Finnish team. You can certainly investigate these preferences – "What makes you so sure Finland would be the most deserving winner of the World Cup?" But I conjecture that, in the end, all it will come down to is "I support Nigeria because I'm Nigerian" or "I support Finland because I'm Finnish." It would be a bit absurd for a committed Finnish fan to approach the Nigerian fan with arguments about why she should transfer her footballing loyalty to Finland. I think there may be a similar pattern in our preferences for different kinds of lives. Contended Australopithecines should be reluctant to give up the known pleasures of an Australopithecine existence for a human existence that they have no knowledge of, and that some self-appointed expert tells them should be better. Humans can certainly respond positively to the obvious embellishments of a posthuman existence. But nothing will rationally compel them, any more than would superior statistics of a Nigerian midfielder compel a Finn to switch loyalties.

Olen: Have you seen artists' representations of Australopithecines? You can't seriously be saying that it would be rational to prefer their lives to ours. Winston, I remember you went through a period of obsessively quoting Shakespeare. Surely you can't be saying that life without Shakespeare could be better than what we have?

Winston: Yes, I moved through my phase of always quoting Shakespeare. But I think that supports my species-relativist point. Of course I love Shakespeare. I'm human! I remember that the biologist Lewis Thomas was asked about messages to send into outer space on the *Voyager* spacecraft to (hopefully!) be heard by extraterrestrial civilizations. He suggested that he would send the complete works of Johann Sebastian Bach but he worried "that would be boasting." Thomas clearly loves Bach as I love Shakespeare but when we move past our human biases we should accept that these are likely to be heard as random noise and pointless sentiments even once perfectly translated into an alien idiolect. It's certainly logically possible that there is intelligent life in HD1, a galaxy identified by astronomers in 2022 and announced as the object most distant from Earth yet detected. It's also logically possible that these beings would experience paroxysms of joy as soon as we play them Bach's B minor Mass. But I nevertheless predict that there will be few Bach fans in HD1.

Sophie: I think you've given us more than enough to think about Winston. Until tomorrow night? But first perhaps I can clarify Winston's opposition to enhancement technologies and radical enhancement. Winston claims to not be a luddite opposed to new technologies and the benefits brought by new tech. His opposition seems to be directed at changes that build them into our human natures. He's happy for new technologies to bring us enormous benefits.

Winston: Yes Sophie, I actually wouldn't mind travelling on a spaceship to Mars, so long as Elon Musk and SpaceX can honour some of their promises about human space travel.

Sophie: So you don't mind being transported to Mars approximately as you are. You just don't want to be turned into a spaceship to get there. The *Bobiverse* future isn't for you. But perhaps the future presented in the *Star Trek* of the 1990s is.

Winston: Yes to go back to our earlier example of the long-division chip. Maybe the long-division chip would bring enormous advantages for those who integrate it into their psyches, but there's something odd about doing that. Why can't we remain approximately as we are and access digital tech that perform these calculations very efficiently but aren't located inside our heads. We can now travel for holidays in distant continents. We do this by getting on board fabulous technologies called passenger jets. Wouldn't there be something a bit odd about someone who came along and presented powered flight as a human enhancement technology? Suppose they suggested grafting wings or jet engines to human bodies. I understand that this is a theme of some of today's superhero movies but I reject it as a programme of human modification. Give me the powered flight without the bionic wings! Give me accurate long division without the brain implants.

Olen: (*angrily*) Winston, I am thoroughly annoyed by the way you and your gorillas have hijacked my beautiful digital techs. I'm going to choose the location of tomorrow night's discussion. Think of it as a final – and decisive – pitch for a radically enhanced future.

Night 9 Three contrasting nightmares about the Age of Human Enhancement

Coffee at SpaceX Headquarters

Olen: All this cynicism about enhancement technologies is killing me! It takes me back to the worst parts of our university disputes. Winston, capitalism is not all bad! There are corrupt capitalists and that's why some of them deservedly end up in jail. But capitalism also lifts people out of poverty. I think that in this Age of Human Enhancement, it promises a much better future for *all* of humanity. We just have to let the tech people do what they excel at. They are business people who understand that companies whose products benefit humanity prosper. The rich will get enhancement technologies first. They will serve as humanity's risk pioneers. Eventually the prices of proven enhancement technologies will come down. The rest of us will get access. Companies in the human enhancement economy will sell first to the rich. But the same forces that now bring smartphones to the poor will make a prosthetic hippocampus available to anyone who wants a better memory. Market forces will carry humanity into enhanced future collectively.

Sophie: This sound suspiciously like a tech version of trickle-down economics. I suspect that your confidence in this future could depend on what you think about the suggestion that enabling the wealthy to further enrich themselves is an effective way to eventually spread that

DOI: 10.4324/9781003321613-9

wealth to the poor. But engaging with that debate will take us too far from our proper focus on the enhancement debate. So, where are we now? It looks like you've chosen this venue to make a final philosophical push for radical human enhancement.

Olen: We're in the Metaverse version of SpaceX's HQ. SpaceX is part of the glorious mission to take humanity into space, to Mars, and beyond. Elon Musk's fortune came from overcoming obstacles blocking electric cars and space exploration. Neuralink – the tech that you are all currently benefitting from – suggests what should happen if we give Musk free rein to apply his tech genius to our human natures. I did tell you that our human natures are failing legacy tech from the Pleistocene, didn't I?

Winston: (*looking sceptical and exasperated*) Yes Olen, you've made that abundantly clear. You're hoping the man who's planning to ferry a million of us to Mars by 2062 is also the man who will radically and promptly remake our natures.

Olen: And why not!

Sophie: Olen, I know that you brought us to SpaceX's HQ to clinch your case for radical human enhancement. But I think we need a different setting to conclude our discussion.

The friends watch as the SpaceX scene slowly fades and is replaced by an altogether more ancient setting.

Olen: (*looking aghast*) What have you done Sophie?!

Sophie: I've shifted location to a venue that is a better fit for our concluding discussion. We are outside the ancient Athens of the 360s BCE. If you look over there you will see a grove of olive trees dedicated to the goddess Athena. This is Plato's Academy.

Eugenie: How is this supposed to help conclude our discussion?

Sophie: We should look back at the Platonic dialogues that were the original inspiration for these discussions about human enhancement. A feature of Platonic dialogues is *aporia*, a state of puzzlement and confusion that characters who start discussion confident that they know what it means to be courageous, pious, or whatever, but are then subjected to a rigorous Socratic inquisition, arrive at. They come to understand that what they thought they knew they don't. Some Platonic dialogues leave readers in a state of *aporia*. In the *Laches* two generals arrive with definite views about what it means to be courageous. Socrates quashes their theories and that's essentially how that dialogue ends. But there are other dialogues in which Socrates takes us beyond a state of *aporia*. He answers some of his own questions. For example, in the *Republic* he tells us what he thinks it means to be just. I think we can view our discussion as more like the *Republic* than the *Laches*.

Olen: So what positive view about human enhancement are we all supposed to take away from this discussion?

Sophie: We haven't arrived at a *single* philosophical theory about human enhancement. Instead we've arrived at something more valuable as we enter the Age of Human Enhancement. There is a difference between the issues that Plato addressed and the issue that we've been addressing. The participants in the *Laches* were engaged in an inquiry into the meaning of courage as it was understood at that time in Athens. The parts of our discussions that have addressed what it means to be enhanced are like this. We arrived at two ways to understand the concept of human enhancement. We agreed that both offer guidance about enhancement technologies. But some of the issues that continue to divide us concern the future development of enhancement technologies. We cannot accurately predict how these techs will progress. This unpredictability means that we do best to preserve all these views about how humanity could or should be transformed by technology.

Olen: (*looking frustrated*) So we conclude our discussion essentially back were we started? This leaves me wondering what the point of all of this was. In the tech industry time is money.

Sophie: We have made significant progress. The Athenian generals conclude the *Laches* with no idea what to say about courage. You all continue to advocate the views you brought to the debate. Olen, you remain an advocate of radical enhancement. Eugenie, you're still a moderate. And Winston, you continue to reject enhancement. I hope that, as others join the discussion, there will be still more views about how humanity should inhabit the Age of Human Enhancement. But I think we don't advocate those views with the same confidence that we did on our first night's discussion. That's a measure of our progress. In the *Apology* Socrates says "I neither know nor think I know." It's dangerous to approach an intrinsically uncertain future with a surfeit of confidence. This means that we need a version of Socrates' attitude as we respond to these uncertainties. As you've been presenting your views about human enhancement, you've also been listening to the views of others and your confidence in your own views has reduced. It can be fun to confidently assert that we know what future enhancement technology will bring. But we would all do well to become less confident about a future that is intrinsically uncertain.

Winston: Perhaps a well-chosen analogy would help.

Sophie: Sure! Olen, the radically enhanced future you've advocated is clearly a logical possibility. But we mustn't forget the lessons from promises that fail to eventuate. Remember that Steven Pinker told us that disease outbreaks don't become pandemics. Viewed from the standpoint of 2018, an indefinitely pandemic-free future was certainly a logical possibility. Moreover, it was certainly a future worth hoping for. But I wonder how much Pinker's optimistic mindset influenced the thinking of politicians as the world confronted the COVID-19 pandemic. How many of them saw images of the empty streets of Wuhan in 2019 and thought that since our technologies and scientific understanding have progressed so much since the 1918 influenza pandemic, we've easily got this. Tetlock refers to "dress to impress forecasting" in which overconfident forecasters offer alluring simplifications of the future when they get on TV or are trying to sell a book. I think that the Age of Human Enhancement will see a lot of dress to impress forecasting about enhancement tech. We should anticipate this and prepare to resist it. Olen, I hope you now wonder what happens if some of your tech forecasts don't pan out.

Olen: I can accept that advice. And in exchange you seem to have accepted the appeal of a radically enhanced future.

Sophie: The more I've listened to your arguments the more I'd like to inhabit the world you describe. But I believe in preparing for a future in which that doesn't happen. We've discussed two kinds of uncertainty about the future of enhancement tech. First, we should insure against a future in which exponential technological progress fails to deliver the wonder techs you are marketing, Olen. There is debate in the integrated circuit industry about how long Moore's Law can continue to deliver its doublings. If tech people are talking that way, it's surely appropriate to doubt whether exponentially improving techs can ever be integrated into the human brain. Winston emphasized a second kind of uncertainty which is about what we value about being human. What if I'm persuaded by the stories transhumanists tell us about a future in which we commit fully to exponentially improving enhancement technologies. I eliminate the capacity for certain feelings because I judge them to be unimportant. But that dismissal stems from a failure to fully grasp how those aspects of our humanity could be valuable. I want us to carry that concern into the Age of Human Enhancement.

Winston: The part of Olen's presentation that most irritated me was when he appealed to Lewis's theory of value on Night 7 to suggest that I value these things for myself even if I am confident I don't. I don't think it's irrational or immoral for me to hope that I eventually die of old age much as the fortunate among us have always done. My historical studies offer plenty of examples of people who led exemplary lives without having to apply exotic enhancement technologies to themselves.

Olen: I'm feeling a bit picked on here!

Sophie: Don't worry, Olen, my mission is to reduce everyone's confidence in their preferred versions of the Age of Human Enhancement. I'm going to test your responses to three different possible futures enhancement tech could make. I've designed a 2100 Age of Human Enhancement scenario specifically for each of you.

Winston: We're listening, Sophie, but could you first tell us what you want to achieve with these stories.

Sophie: I want you to accept that if the Age of Human Enhancement turns out in a way you don't expect that you would concede that you were significantly, if not entirely, mistaken about whether and how we should apply enhancement technologies to ourselves. You need not be reduced to the philosophical defeat of *aporia* to make this concession. You can certainly continue to vigorously argue that things won't turn out in the way my scenarios present.

Three year 2100 human enhancement what-ifs

Sophie: Here's your 2100 scenario Olen. (*Text appears between the friends.*)

Olen's Nightmare: The years leading up to 2100 saw rapid improvement in enhancement technologies. There was widespread recognition that the most efficient path to a radically enhanced future was not by editing human genes or by designing nootropics but by applying exponentially improving digital technologies directly to human brains and bodies. The first generations of these techs were effective but very expensive, so expensive that they were available only to the billionaire class. The beneficiaries of these improvements insisted that the digital enhancement techs that rich enjoy would soon be available to all. And they do get cheaper. But the logic of exponential improvement meant the primitively enhanced poor were left farther and farther behind. The poor found that by the time they got access to a new enhancement tech, the rich had already moved on to much more powerful techs. A class of humans classified as "the left behind" now includes the unenhanced but also the primitively enhanced, those with obsolete enhancement techs. The enhanced elite feel no more strongly connected to the left behind than they do to gorillas clinging on in vestigial habitats. Among some of the radically enhanced elite there are increasing expressions of doubt about the path our species has taken. There is an increasingly popular "back to human nature" movement among the most enhanced. But there is a recognition that the technologically simple pleasures of an unenhanced human nature are no longer available to them. They are as available to the radically enhanced as were the putative pleasures of pre-Neolithic subsistence farming to the city dwellers of the early twenty-first century.

Olen: I strongly doubt that this will happen.
Sophie: That's not at issue here. This is a logically possible scenario compatible with the laws of physics. If Olen's Nightmare did come to pass would you change your philosophical view about human enhancement?
Olen: I think I would. Now can you stop picking on me?
Sophie: Sure. Here's a story for Eugenie. (*Text appears between the friends.*)

Eugenie's Nightmare: The years leading up to 2100 saw rapid improvement in enhancement technologies. In the middle decades of the twenty-first century a decision was made to reject the path of integrating digital technologies into human brains and bodies. Several scandals cast the idea of augmenting human psyches and physiologies with silicon technology into significant disrepute. The greatest outrage was the hacking of a prosthetic hippocampus causing its bearer to detonate a bomb on a transatlantic flight. Companies manufacturing these implants insisted that they could improve the security of these devices. But among the voting public in the most technologically advanced democracies, there were fears about designers of the latest chips secreting "zombie switches" into their devices. These fears were aggravated by a recognition that some of these chips were manufactured in nations with hostile foreign policies, leading to a panic about cyber Manchurian candidates. The United Nations imposed and enforced a ban on the development of neuroprostheses for the purpose of human enhancement. Public interest in enhancement switched to genetic technologies. Rich world governments significantly liberalized the editing of human genomes. Some prospective parents adopted the attitude of risk pioneers on behalf of their future children editing a wide variety of the genes that influence intelligence. There were many stories about genetic engineering experiments that went horribly wrong leaving children with disfigured psyches and physiologies. Wealthy parents became reluctant to apply unproven gene edits to their children's genomes. So they paid poor people to test them on their children. Liberal democratic governments responded with legal prohibitions, but many wealthy parents adapted by offshoring their experiments in genetic enhancement to poorer nations. The United Nations failed to intervene. Today thoughtful wealthy parents justify the practice of paying the poor to test genetic enhancements by accepting that it is exploitative, but reasoning that this exploitation is mutually beneficial. Payments to the poor who offer their children to be genetic enhancement guinea pigs lift some out of poverty. Shrewd parents arrange for the wealthy to cover their children's medical expenses for experiments in genetic enhancement that turn out badly. Over time a stock of safe genetic enhancements has emerged. But this system of mutually beneficial exploitation is ongoing as new potential enhancements are proposed and widening wealth inequality increases the pressure on the poor to test the genetic enhancements demanded by the rich. Some of wealthy are morally enhanced too. They worry about the injustices of the Age of Human Enhancement but feel powerless to do anything about them.

Sophie: What do you make of that, Eugenie?

Eugenie: It sounds like scaremongering to me. The liberal democratic states of the near future will have many means to prevent these outcomes.

Sophie: No surprises that you're confident about that. But what if a crystal ball revealed that this was the future made by enhancement technologies? Would you question your support for the liberal approach?

Eugenie: Well, if you put it that way, I guess I would.

Sophie: Don't worry, Winston, I haven't forgotten about you. Here's your story. (*Text appears between the friends.*)

Winston's Nightmare: The years leading up to 2100 saw rapid improvement in enhancement technologies. As these technologies were released there were fears of abuse. This prompted strict and effective oversight. Liberal governments were successful in balancing individuals' rights to apply a wide range of enhancement technologies to themselves and their children and the need for social solidarity. Today governments tax the latest enhancement technologies enabling them to subsidize access for the poor. The poor do not receive the latest enhancements but human enhancement support schemes nevertheless ensure that the cognitive gaps between rich and poor are not great. The United Nations works with the World Health Organization to offer these enhancements throughout the poor world. Initially there were fears about the impact of radical enhancement on relationships. But couples who approach enhancement facilities together generally find that going through the enhancement process as a couple means that they emerge with their relationships transformed but intact. The radically cognitively enhanced are much more intelligent than unenhanced humans but they still feel human and express a sense of kinship with the unenhanced. The dominant sentiment of the Age of Human Enhancement is one of celebrating diversity and the many different ways to be human. The posthumans of 2100 have a variety of skin colours and are able to easily change them to express solidarity with different pre-Age of Human Enhancement populations. The posthumans understand that their biological parts connect them to ancestral human populations from all over the globe. However, they increasingly identify with the parts of their psyches remade by tech. There remain some unenhanced humans. There is widespread agreement among morally enhanced posthumans that they are obliged to use their superior intelligence to ensure the flourishing of these vestigial unenhanced human populations. There is a collective sense of triumph about how our species is traversing the Age of Human Enhancement.

Olen: I like the way Winston's Nightmare is when everything turns out great. You really are personally invested in your theories aren't you, Winston?

Winston: You won't be surprised to hear that I think this is unlikely to happen.

Sophie: Yes, but that's not the key issue here. My story violates no law of physics or logic. If it did come to pass would you change your mind about radical enhancement, and enhancement in general?

Winston: Remember that I'm the one whose rejection of enhancement tech means I don't plan to be around in 2100. But if that's the way 2100 turns out then I expect my doubts to be dismissed much in the way we now view people who argue against the theory of evolution. But that doesn't invalidate my current opposition to enhancement tech in the early twenty-first century.

Sophie: Time to draw our discussion to a close. I'm confident I have enough now to commence my thesis. I've learned a great deal from your disagreements and occasional agreements. The most important thing as we advance into the Age of Human Enhancement is to keep talking. The coming decades will bring a wide variety of enhancement techs. We must be careful to listen to the views of people outside of the coming enhancement tech industry. Speaking as an aspiring academic philosopher I would like to hear more from poets, storytellers, and painters. They may not know much about tech. But they do understand the human condition. They give the clearest possible expression of what it means to be human and what's worth preserving about our humanity. We need to hear from them to not lose our connection with what really matters about being human. I worry that in our enhanced future the sentiments expressed in Toni Morrison's *Beloved* trilogy or by the poet Li Bai may be as meaningful to us as they are to the alien inhabitants of that HD1 galaxy that we speculated about last night. Let's read as much Morrison and Shakespeare as we can before it's too late.

Olen: Duly noted. I hope my neural lace's sneaky enhancement of your cognitive faculties hasn't already denied you these very human pleasures.

Sophie: I think they are still within reach of me. I just used your wonder tech to display Emily Dickinson's poem *Each Life Converges to some Centre*.

Each Life Converges to some Centre –
Expressed – or still –
Exists in every Human Nature
A Goal –

Embodied scarcely to itself …

I still get this. Perhaps this is selfish, but I hope that my possibly radically enhanced descendants still get it too.

Annotated bibliography

The characters in these *Dialogues on Human Enhancement* discuss a variety of issues in what is a fast-expanding philosophical literature on the ethics of applying enhancement technologies to human nature. In what follows I list readings on the philosophy of human enhancement that should empower readers to contribute to the debate. I hope readers are inspired to use them continue lines of discussion when the debate seems to trail off in the dialogues. There many important philosophical contributions that are missing from the following list. I encourage students to add characters to the dialogues that express these omitted contributions. How might Olen, Winston, Eugenie, or Sophie respond if you raise an enhancement ethics issue with them that they thoughtlessly overlook?

The following list commences with general introductions to the debate. Reading pertinent to each section of the dialogue appear under headings for that section. Readers will find many entries from the *Stanford Encyclopedia of Philosophy*. This is an especially useful starting point for serious students of philosophy.

General introductions to the philosophy of human enhancement

GENERAL INTRODUCTIONS TO THE DEBATE ABOUT HUMAN ENHANCEMENT

Anomaly, Jonathan, *Creating Future People: The Ethics of Genetic Enhancement* (Routledge, 2020).

Juengst, Eric and Daniel Moseley, "Human Enhancement", *The Stanford Encyclopedia of Philosophy* (Summer 2019 Edition), Edward N. Zalta (ed.), URL = https://plato.stanford.edu/archives/sum2019/entries/enhancement/.
Savulescu, Julian and Nick Bostrom, *Human Enhancement* (Oxford University Press, 2009).

ADVOCATES OF HUMAN ENHANCEMENT

Buchanan, Allen, *Better than Human: The Promise and Perils of Enhancing Ourselves* (Oxford University Press, 2011).
Buchanan, Allen, *Beyond Humanity?: The Ethics of Biomedical Enhancement* (Oxford University Press, 2011).
Harris, John, *Enhancing Evolution: The Ethical Case for Making Better People* (Princeton University Press, 2007).

CRITICS OF HUMAN ENHANCEMENT

Diéguez, Antonio, *Cuerpos Inadecuados* (Herder, 2019).
Fukuyama, Francis, *Our Posthuman Future: Consequences of the Biotechnology Revolution* (Picador, 2003).
Hauskeller, Michael, *Better Humans?: Understanding the Enhancement Project* (Routledge, 2013).
Kass, Leon, *Life Liberty & the Defense of Dignity: The Challenge for Bioethics* (Encounter Books, 2003).
Sandel, Michael, *The Price of Perfection: Ethics in the Age of Genetic Engineering* (Harvard University Press, 2007).

Night 1: What should we say about gene-edited twins who may have been enhanced?

THE HE JIANKUI AFFAIR

Juengst, Eric, Gail Henderson, Rebecca Walker, John Conley, Douglas MacKay, Karen Meagher, et al., "Is Enhancement the Price of Prevention in Human Gene Editing?", *The CRISPR Journal*, 1(6), (2018).
Greely, Henry, "CRISPR'd babies: human germline genome editing in the 'He Jiankui affair'", *Journal of Law and the Biosciences*, 6(1), (2019).
McIntyre, Alison, "Doctrine of Double Effect", *The Stanford Encyclopedia of Philosophy* (Spring 2019 Edition), Edward N. Zalta (ed.), URL = https://plato.stanford.edu/archives/spr2019/entries/double-effect/.

THE IMPORTANCE OF BEING REASONABLE ABOUT AN ESSENTIALLY UNCERTAIN FUTURE

Pinker, Steven, *Enlightenment Now: The Case for Reason, Science, Humanism, and Progress* (Viking, 2018).
Tetlock, Philip and Dan Gardner, *Superforecasting: The Art and Science of Prediction* (Crown Publishers, 2015).

Night 2: Enhancement technologies, doping athletes, and the meaning of human enhancement

WHAT ARE ENHANCEMENT TECHNOLOGIES?

Bird, Alexander and Emma Tobin, "Natural Kinds", *The Stanford Encyclopedia of Philosophy* (Spring 2022 Edition), Edward N. Zalta (ed.), URL = https://plato.stanford.edu/archives/spr2022/entries/natural-kinds/.

Moseley, Daniel and Christina Murray, "Biomedical Technology and the Ethics of Enhancement" in G. Robson and J. Tsou (eds.), *Technology Ethics: A Philosophical Introduction and Readings* (Routledge, 2023).

DID BEN JOHNSON REALLY CHEAT AT THE 1988 SEOUL OLYMPICS?

Devine, John William and Francisco Javier Lopez Frias, "Philosophy of Sport", *The Stanford Encyclopedia of Philosophy* (Fall 2020 Edition), Edward N. Zalta (ed.), URL = https://plato.stanford.edu/archives/fall2020/entries/sport/.

Savulescu, Julian, Bennett Foddy, and Matthew Clayton, "Why we should allow performance enhancing drugs in sport", *British Journal of Sports Medicine*, 38(6), (2003).

Miah, Andy, *Genetically Modified Athletes: Biomedical Ethics, Gene Doping and Sport* (Routledge, 2004).

Murray, Tom, *Ethics, Genetics and the Future of Sport: Implications of Genetic Modification and Genetic Selection* (Georgetown University Press, 2009).

Night 3: From Francis Galton's eugenics to liberal eugenics

FRANCIS GALTON AND EUGENICS

Anomaly, Johnathan, "Defending Eugenics: From cryptic choice to conscious selection", *Monash Bioethics Review* 35, (2018).

de Melo-Martin, Inmaculada and Sara Goering, "Eugenics", *The Stanford Encyclopedia of Philosophy* (Summer 2022 Edition), Edward N. Zalta (ed.), URL = https://plato.stanford.edu/archives/sum2022/entries/eugenics/.

Galton, Francis, *Inquiries into Human Faculty and its Development* (Macmillan and Co, 1883).

Kevles, Daniel, *In the Name of Eugenics: Genetics and the Uses of Human Heredity* (Harvard University Press, 1998).

Paul, Diane, *Controlling Human Heredity: 1865 To the Present* (Humanities Books, 1995).

Wilson, Robert, "Eugenics, Disability, and Bioethics" in Joel Reynolds and Christine Weiseler (eds.), *The Disability Bioethics Reader* (Routledge, 2022).

THE ETHICAL FIX OF "LIBERAL" EUGENICS

Agar, Nicholas, *Liberal Eugenics: In Defence of Human Enhancement* (John Wiley & Sons, 2004).

Blackford, Russell, *Humanity Enhanced: Genetic Choice and the Challenge for Liberal Democracies* (MIT Press, 2014).

Habermas, Jürgen, *The Future of Human Nature* (Polity, 2003).

Robertson, John, *Children of Choice: Freedom and the New Reproductive Technologies* (Princeton University Press, 1994).

Sparrow, Robert, "Liberalism and Eugenics", *Australasian Journal of Philosophy*, 89(3), (2011).

A THOUGHT EXPERIMENT INVOLVING AN ENHANCED HIMMLER

Bennett, Jonathan, "The Conscience of Huckleberry Finn", *Philosophy* 49, (1974).

WHAT IS PROCREATIVE LIBERTY?

Blackford, Russell, *Humanity Enhanced: Genetic Choice and the Challenge for Liberal Democracies* (MIT Press, 2014)

Brake, Elizabeth and Joseph Millum, "Parenthood and Procreation", *The Stanford Encyclopedia of Philosophy* (Spring 2022 Edition), Edward N. Zalta (ed.), URL = https://plato.stanford.edu/archives/spr2022/entries/parenthood/.

Robertson, John, *Children of Choice: Freedom and the New Reproductive Technologies* (Princeton University Press, 1994).

IS HUMAN ENHANCEMENT A THREAT TO EQUALITY?

Buchanan, Allen, D. W. Brock, N. Daniels, and D. Wikler, *From Chance to Choice: Genetics and Justice* (Cambridge University Press, 2000).

Savulescu, Julian, "Procreative Beneficence: Why we should Select the Best Children", *Bioethics* 15, (2001).

Silver, Lee, *Remaking Eden: How Genetic Engineering and Cloning Will Transform the American* Family (Ecco, 2007).

WILL HUMAN ENHANCEMENT END SEX?

Sparrow, Robert. "Human enhancement and sexual dimorphism" *Bioethics*, 26(9), (2012).

IS LIBERAL EUGENICS JUST SHIT STIRRING?

Agar, Nicholas, "One the Moral Obligation to Stop Shit-stirring" *Psyche*, 15 December, 2020, URL = https://psyche.co/ideas/on-the-moral-obligation-to-stop-shit-stirring

Agar, Nicholas, "Confessions of a Philosophical Shit-stirrer" *ABC*, 1 December, 2021, URL = www.abc.net.au/religion/confessions-of-a-philosophical-shit-stirrer/13611942

Frankfurt, Harry, *On Bullshit* (Princeton University Press, 2005).

Night 4: Radical versus moderate enhancement and cognition

DIFFERENCES BETWEEN LIBERAL EUGENICS AND RADICAL
ENHANCEMENT

Agar, Nicholas, *Humanity's End: Why we should Reject Radical Enhancement* (MIT Press, 2010).
Agar, Nicholas, *Truly Human Enhancement: A Philosophical Defense of Limits* (MIT Press, 2013).

SHOULD WE BECOME POSTHUMAN?

Agar, Nicholas, "What Does it Mean to be Human, Prehuman, or Posthuman?", *Journal of Posthuman Studies*, 5(1), (2021).
Bostrom, Nick, "Human Genetic Enhancements: A Transhumanist Perspective", *The Journal of Value Inquiry*, 37(4), (2003).
Bostrom, Nick, "Why I Want to be a Posthuman When I Grow Up" in Bert Gordijn and Ruth Chadwick (eds.), *Medical Enhancement and Posthumanity* (Springer, 2008).
Hayles, N. Katherine, *How We Became Posthuman: Virtual Bodies in Cybernetics, Literature, and Informatics* (University of Chicago Press, 1999).
Hughes, James, *Citizen Cyborg: Why Democratic Societies Must Respond to the Redesigned Human of the Future* (Westview Press, 2004).
Leakey, Richard, *Origins Reconsidered: In Search of What Makes Us Human* (Little, Brown, 1992).
Levin, Susan, *Posthuman Bliss? The Failed Promise of Transhumanism* (Oxford University Press, 2021).
Roduit, Johann, *The Case for Perfection: Ethics in the Age of Human Enhancement* (Peter Lang, 2016).
Sorgner, Stefan Lorenz, *We Have Always Been Cyborgs: Digital Data, Gene Technologies, and an Ethics of Transhumanism* (Bristol University Press, 2023).
"The Transhumanist FAQ: revised version 2.1", URL = https://nickbostrom.com

WHAT IS EXPONENTIAL TECHNOLOGICAL PROGRESS?

Kurzweil, Ray, *The Singularity is Near: When Humans Transcend Biology* (Viking Books, 2005)

CAN WE HAVE RADICALLY ENHANCED COGNITIVE POWERS?

Sniekers, Suzanne, Sven Stringer, Kyoko Watanabe, Philip R. Jansen, Jonathan R. I. Coleman, Eva Krapohl, Erdogan Taskesen, et al. "Genome-wide association meta-analysis of 78,308 individuals identifies new loci and genes influencing human intelligence", *Nature Genetics*, 49(7), (2017).

Night 5: SENS and radical life extension

ADICALLY EXTENDED LIFESPANS

Davis, John, *New Methuselahs: The Ethics of Life Extension* (MIT Press, 2018).
de Grey, Aubrey and Michael Rae, *Ending Aging: The Rejuvenation Breakthroughs that Could Reverse Human Aging in our Lifetime* (St Martin's Press, 2007).
Linden, Ingemar Patrick, *The Case against Death* (MIT Press, 2022).
Samuel Scheffler, *Death and the Afterlife* (Oxford University Press, 2016)

CAN *SENS* MAKE HUMANS NEGLIGIBLY SENESCENT?

Wadman, Meredith, "Antiaging scientist found to have sexually harassed young women", *ScienceInsider*, 13 September, 2021, URL = www.science.org/content/article/antiaging-scientist-found-have-sexually-harassed-young-women

MIGHT *SENS* ACTUALLY SLOW PROGRESS TOWARD AN ENHANCED FUTURE?

Michael Shnayerson, *Boom: Mad Money, Mega Dealers, and the Rise of Contemporary Art* (PublicAffairs, 2019)

WHY ADVOCATES OF MODERATE ENHANCEMENT MIGHT PREFER GENE EDITING TO ENHANCEMENT BY DIGITAL TECH

Tsien, Joe Z., "Building a Brainier Mouse", *Scientific American*, 282(4), (April 2000).

Night 6: Enhanced moods and morality

Haybron, Dan, "Happiness", *The Stanford Encyclopedia of Philosophy* (Summer 2020 Edition), Edward N. Zalta (ed.), URL = https://plato.stanford.edu/archives/sum2020/entries/happiness/.

HAPPY-PEOPLE-PILLS FOR ALL?

Walker, Mark, *Happy-People-Pills for All* (Wiley-Blackwell, 2013).

CAN WE CONTROL EXPONENTIALLY IMPROVING DIGITAL TECHNOLOGIES?

Douglas, Thomas, "Moral Enhancement", *Journal of Applied Philosophy*, 25(3), (2008).
Harris, John, *How to be Good? The Possibility of Moral Enhancement* (Oxford University Press, 2016)
Jotterand, Fabrice, *The Unfit Brain and the Limits of Moral Bioenhancement* (Palgrave Macmillan, 2022).

Persson, Ingmar and Julian Savulescu, *Unfit for the Future: The Need for Moral Enhancement* (Oxford University Press, 2012).

Weber, Elke, "What shapes perceptions of climate change?",*Climate Change*, 1, (2010).

Wiseman, Harris, *The Myth of the Moral Brain: The Limits of Moral Enhancement* (MIT Press, 2016)

Zak, Paul, *The Moral Molecule: How Trust Works* (Dutton, 2012).

Night 7: How do we decide which aspects of human nature to preserve?

THE MEANING OF THE LUDDITES

Thompson, E. P., *The Making of the English Working Class* (Vintage Books, 1963).

WHAT WOULD WE DO TO AVOID EXTINCTION?

Rakić, Vojin, "Voluntary moral enhancement and the survival-at-any-cost bias", *Journal of Medical Ethics*, 40(4), (2014).

SHOULD WE WANT THE THINGS WE BELIEVE OUR RADICALLY ENHANCED FUTURE SELVES MIGHT WANT?

Smith, Michael, David Lewis and Mark Johnston, "Dispositional Theories of Value", *Aristotelian Society*, Supplementary Volume 63(1), (1989).

FROM SURVEILLANCE CAPITALISM TO ENHANCEMENT CAPITALISM?

Shoshana Zuboff, *The Age of Surveillance Capitalism: The Fight for a Human Future at the New Frontier of Power* (Profile Books, 2019)

PHILOSOPHICAL UNCERTAINTY ABOUT WHAT IT MEANS TO BE HUMAN

Hudson, Maui, Ahuriri-Driscoll, A., Lea, M., and Lea, R. "Whakapapa: A Foundation for Genetic Research", *Journal of Bioethical Inquiry*, 4, (2007).

Night 8: A species relativist rejection of radical enhancement

IS RADICAL ENHANCEMENT A TRANSFORMATIVE CHANGE?

Bykvist, Krister, "Review of L. A. Paul, Transformative Experience", *Notre Dame Philosophical Reviews*, URL = https://ndpr.nd.edu/news/61570-transformative-experience/

Paul, Laurie, *Transformative Experience* (Oxford University Press, 2014).

A KIND OF SPECIES RELATIVISM?

Baghramian, Maria and J. Adam Carter, "Relativism", *The Stanford Encyclopedia of Philosophy* (Spring 2022 Edition), Edward N. Zalta (ed.), URL = https://plato.stanford.edu/archives/spr2022/entries/relativism/.
Gowans, Chris, "Moral Relativism", *The Stanford Encyclopedia of Philosophy* (Spring 2021 Edition), Edward N. Zalta (ed.), URL = https://plato.stanford.edu/archives/spr2021/entries/moral-relativism/.

Night 9: Three contrasting nightmares about the Age of Human Enhancement

THREE YEAR 2100 HUMAN ENHANCEMENT WHAT-IFS

Zwolinski, Matt, Benjamin Ferguson, and Alan Wertheimer, "Exploitation", *The Stanford Encyclopedia of Philosophy* (Winter 2022 Edition), Edward N. Zalta & Uri Nodelman (eds.), URL = https://plato.stanford.edu/archives/win2022/entries/exploitation/.

Index

For Product Safety Concerns and Information please contact our
EU representative GPSR@taylorandfrancis.com Taylor & Francis
Verlag GmbH, Kaufingerstraße 24, 80331 München, Germany